BASIC GUIDE TO DENTAL PROCEDURES

Third Edition

Carole Hollins

General Dental Practitioner
Member of the British Dental Association
Former Chairman and presiding examiner for the National Examining Board
for Dental Nurses

WILEY Blackwell

Registered Offices
John Wiley & Sons, Inc., 111 River Street, Hoboken, NJ 07030, USA
John Wiley & Sons Ltd, The Atrium, Southern Gate, Chichester, West Sussex, PO19 8SQ, UK

For details of our global editorial offices, customer services, and more information about Wiley products visit us at www.wiley.com.

Wiley also publishes its books in a variety of electronic formats and by print-on-demand. Some content that appears in standard print versions of this book may not be available in other formats.

Library of Congress Cataloging-in-Publication Data
Names: Hollins, Carole, author.
Title: Basic guide to dental procedures / Carole Hollins.
Description: Third edition. | Hoboken, NJ : Wiley-Blackwell, 2024. |
   Includes index.
Identifiers: LCCN 2024000366 (print) | LCCN 2024000367 (ebook) |
   ISBN 9781394187874 (paperback) | ISBN 9781394187881 (adobe pdf) |
   ISBN 9781394187898 (epub)
Subjects: MESH: Dentistry–methods | Dental Assistants | Handbook
Classification: LCC RK56 (print) | LCC RK56 (ebook) | NLM WU 49 | DDC
   617.6–dc23/eng/20240318
LC record available at https://lccn.loc.gov/2024000366
LC ebook record available at https://lccn.loc.gov/2024000367

Cover Design: Wiley
Cover Image: Courtesy of Carole Hollins

Set in 9/11pt SabonLTStd by Straive, Pondicherry, India
SKY10071663_040424

Contents

How to use this book

As the title suggests, the book has been written as an introductory guide to the more usual dental procedures carried out in a modern dental practice. It does not attempt to explain the full theoretical and clinical technique behind these procedures; rather, it aims to give a sufficient overview of them, with the use of 'before and after' colour photographs and various illustrations to hopefully make the book useful for helping to explain certain dental procedures to patients and also to unqualified dental nurses undergoing their primary training in dental nursing. In this third edition, each chapter has been updated as necessary in line with the latest dental techniques and materials available to the profession. A new chapter relating to treatment under conscious sedation has been included for the benefit of the patients and is also of relevance to the dental nurse in the United Kingdom, as their role in assisting during the treatment of patients under conscious sedation is an extended duty.

However, the main readership is envisaged to be dental care professionals, especially those unqualified or inexperienced dental nurses who may not have access to viewing many of the procedures described, as many practices continue to specialise in providing dental care only in certain areas of dentistry. It should be used, then, in conjunction with the excellent textbooks already available for dental nurse training, where more detail of instruments and materials used, more in-depth clinical information and other underpinning knowledge are provided. By popular request, photographic examples of the instruments and materials, which may be required for various procedures, have been retained in this edition, and while the images used provide guidance for those undertaking OSCE-style training and assessment, they are not intended to be exhaustive in their content.

The text in each section is laid out to explain the reasons behind the treatment described, the relevant dental background, the basics of how each procedure is carried out and any aftercare information necessary. It is beyond the remit of the book to cover every current technique in every dental discipline discussed, so it is hoped that the text provides at least the basic information required for the reader to gain an understanding of the procedure, before seeking a greater depth of knowledge elsewhere.

The inclusion and expansion of information on extended duties for dental nurses in this edition, as in the previous edition, is of particular relevance to the United Kingdom-based readership. Examples have been given throughout the chapter of the type and extent of 'in-house' training that may be provided in a broad selection of these duties, as well as examples of suggested recording sheets that may be used to provide evidence of monitoring and competency in various of the necessary skills discussed. It is hoped that the information provided will help UK dental practices train and extend the useful skills of its workforce in an effort to develop their dental team and widen their provision of dental services for the ultimate benefit of their patients.

Wherever possible, the correct dental terminology has been adhered to, but as the dental knowledge of the expected readership will vary widely, a glossary of terms has been updated again and included to clarify certain definitions in the context to which they have been referred to in the text.

Chapter 1

Preventive techniques

REASON FOR PROCEDURE

Preventive techniques are aimed at reducing a patient's risk of experiencing the onset of dental caries in teeth, thereby helping to maintain the dental health of a patient.

The two procedures discussed are:

- Application of fissure sealants
- Application of topical fluorides – full mouth or specific teeth

BACKGROUND INFORMATION OF PROCEDURE – FISSURE SEALANTS

Any surface area of a tooth that cannot be cleaned easily by the patient can allow food debris, and ultimately plaque, to accumulate there and allow caries to develop by acting as a stagnation area. Plaque is the term used to describe the soft, sticky film that forms in the mouth whenever food is ingested and is composed of food debris and oral bacteria. Patients usually clean their teeth by brushing, flossing, using other interdental cleaning aids, mouth washing, or any combination of these techniques.

The usual sites that can act as stagnation areas are the occlusal pits and fissures of posterior teeth (Figure 1.1), especially the first permanent molars which erupt at around 6 years of age. Fissures are seen on the occlusal (biting) surface of the teeth, while pits are usually seen on the buccal (cheek side) of the teeth.

These teeth are particularly prone to caries because:

- They are the least accessible teeth for cleaning, being at the back of the young patient's mouth (they erupt behind the deciduous set of teeth).
- They erupt at an age (around 6 years old) when a good oral hygiene regime is unlikely to have been developed, so may be cleaned poorly by the patient initially.

Basic Guide to Dental Procedures, Third Edition. Carole Hollins.
© 2024 John Wiley & Sons Ltd. Published 2024 by John Wiley & Sons Ltd.

PREVENTIVE TECHNIQUES

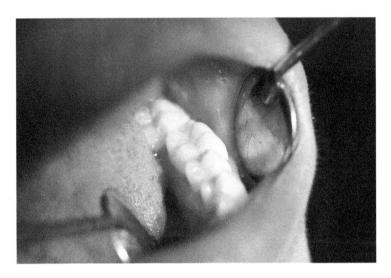

Figure 1.1 Occlusal fissures of lower left molar tooth

- Younger patients often have a diet containing more sugar than adults, as the concept of dietary control will not yet be appreciated.

DETAILS OF PROCEDURE – FISSURE SEALANTS

The occlusal pit or fissure needs to be eliminated to prevent it from acting as a stagnation area and allowing plaque to accumulate there, and this is achieved by filling in the inaccessible depth with a sealant material.

The materials used are either unfilled resins, flowable composites, glass ionomer cement, or a combination of these latter two materials (known as a compomer).

The usual instruments and materials that may be laid out for a fissure sealant procedure are shown in Figure 1.2.

TECHNIQUE:

- The operator and the patient wear suitable personal protective equipment
- The tooth is kept isolated from saliva contamination, as materials will not adhere to the tooth when it is wet
- Isolation techniques include the use of cotton wool rolls and low-speed suction techniques using a saliva ejector (Figure 1.3).
- The occlusal fissures and pits are chemically roughened with acid etch to allow the microscopic bonding of the sealant material to the enamel
- The etch is washed off, and the tooth is dried; the etched surface will appear chalky white
- Unfilled resin is run into the etched areas to seal the fissures or pits and then locked into the enamel structure by setting with a curing lamp
- If any demineralisation of the fissure is present, one of the alternative flowable materials listed above is used to replace the demineralised enamel surface

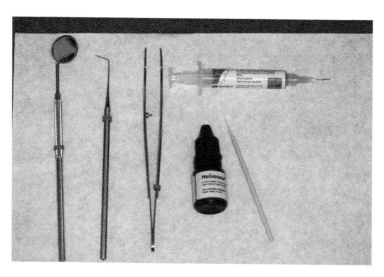

Figure 1.2 Fissure sealant instruments and materials

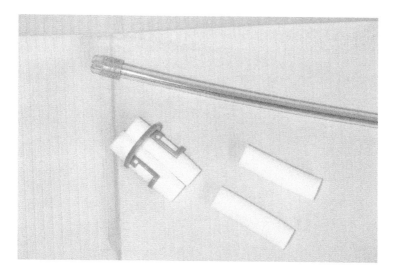

Figure 1.3 Tooth isolation techniques

BACKGROUND INFORMATION OF PROCEDURE – TOPICAL FLUORIDE

Other areas of the teeth that are very difficult to clean are the points where they have contact with each other in the dental arch – the interproximal (interdental) areas.

There are certain oral health products available specifically for cleaning these areas, such as dental floss and interdental brushes, but they require a certain amount of dexterity and determination by the patient to be used effectively.

All fluoridated toothpastes provide some protection of these areas from dental caries ('tooth decay'), but some patients require additional full mouth fluoride protection by the professional application of a topical fluoride varnish or gel.

They are:

- Children and vulnerable adults with high caries rates
- Children undergoing fixed orthodontic treatment (fixed braces)
- Adults with increased risk factors for caries, such as a heavily restored dentition, persistent dry mouth due to medications or medical conditions, and so on
- Physically disabled patients who are unable to achieve a good level of oral hygiene due to the limitations of their physical disability
- Medically compromised patients for whom tooth extractions are too dangerous to be carried out (haemophiliacs, patients with some heart defects)

DETAILS OF PROCEDURE – FULL MOUTH TOPICAL FLUORIDE APPLICATION

A high concentration of fluoride is required to be applied to the interproximal areas that are viscous enough not to be washed away quickly by saliva so that it can be taken into the enamel structure of the tooth during contact, thereby making it more resistant to caries. The usual material used is a sticky fluoride varnish or gel, such as one of those shown in Figure 1.4.

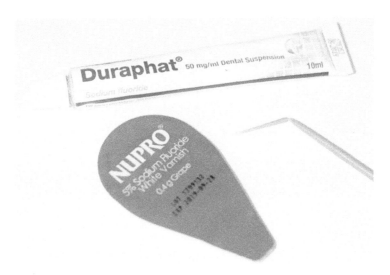

Figure 1.4 Examples of topical fluoride varnishes for professional application

TECHNIQUE:

- The operator and the patient wear suitable personal protective equipment
- The teeth are polished with a pumice slurry to remove any plaque present and allow the maximum tooth contact with the fluoride
- The polish is thoroughly washed off, and the teeth are dried
- Adequate soft tissue retraction and moisture control are provided by the dental nurse so that the dry tooth surfaces are accessible and the gel will not be displaced by accident during the procedure
- The viscous fluoride gel is manually applied to all available surfaces of each tooth, using one or more applicator buds and treating one arch at a time
- Previously, an alternative application technique involved the use of preformed trays for each arch, which were loaded with the fluoride varnish before insertion and then held in place by the operator for some time to allow the fluoride to become incorporated into the enamel surface. The aforementioned manual application technique tends to be better tolerated by the patient

DETAILS OF PROCEDURE – SPECIFIC TOOTH TOPICAL FLUORIDE APPLICATION

In some patients, individual teeth may show signs of previous acid attack from certain foods and drinks, such as a 'brown spot' lesion on the enamel surface (Figure 1.5). Other patients may have an area of gingival recession or toothbrush abrasion present, either of which exposes the root surface of a tooth to dietary acids and sugars, therefore making it vulnerable to attack by dental caries (see Figure 5.9). These specific areas can be protected by the direct application of a localised fluoride varnish, such as those shown in Figure 1.4, using a technique similar to that of a full-mouth application as described earlier.

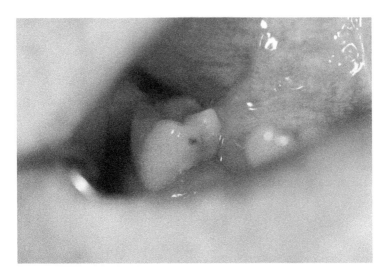

Figure 1.5 Brown spot lesion indicating previous enamel damage

Chapter 2

Oral hygiene instruction

REASON FOR PROCEDURE

Oral hygiene instruction is given to patients to ensure that they are maximising their efforts to remove plaque from their teeth and gingival margins to minimise the damage caused by dental caries and periodontal disease, respectively.

Dietary advice is also given to help patients avoid foods and drinks that are particularly damaging to their teeth – those high in refined sugars or those that are acidic.

When the advice is correctly followed on a regular basis, the patients can enjoy a well-cared-for and pain-free mouth, as well as avoid the expense of reparative dental treatment.

The procedures discussed are:

- Use of disclosing agents
- Toothbrushing instruction
- Interdental cleaning instruction
- Dietary advice to reduce the risk of dental caries

BACKGROUND INFORMATION OF PROCEDURE – DISCLOSING AGENTS

Disclosing agents are harmless vegetable dyes supplied in liquid or tablet form and in various colours, usually red or blue (Figure 2.1). Alternatively, a similar disclosing action can be achieved by swilling the mouth with a solution of food colourant liquid (such as those used to colour cake icing).

The disclosing agents act by staining any plaque on the tooth surface to their colour (Figure 2.2), thus making it far easier to show the presence and location of the plaque to the patient, as plaque is normally a creamy white colour and may be difficult for the patient to see otherwise (Figure 2.3).

Basic Guide to Dental Procedures, Third Edition. Carole Hollins.
© 2024 John Wiley & Sons Ltd. Published 2024 by John Wiley & Sons Ltd.

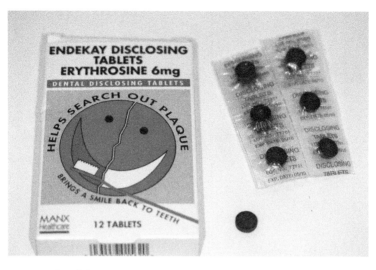

Figure 2.1 Examples of disclosing tablets

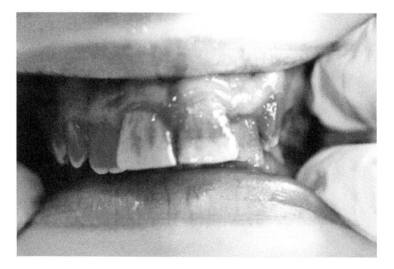

Figure 2.2 Disclosed teeth showing the presence and extent of plaque build-up

Once stained, suitable oral hygiene instructions can be given to remove the plaque effectively. The dyes stain the plaque present on the teeth and gums, but not the teeth themselves, nor any restorations. However, they will also stain any plaque present on other soft tissues, such as the tongue – an area that few patients would think to brush as a matter of routine. Showing the presence of stained plaque in these areas helps persuade patients to carefully brush them routinely as part of their oral hygiene regime.

ORAL HYGIENE INSTRUCTION

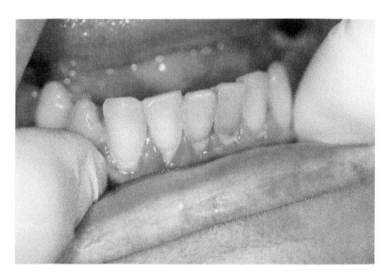

Figure 2.3 Appearance of undisclosed gingival plaque

DETAILS OF PROCEDURE – DISCLOSING AGENTS

The agents can initially be used at the practice by the oral health team so that the correct problem areas can be identified and suitable cleaning advice can be given. The patient can then use the agents at home to check their progress on a regular basis. The most common agents used are disclosing tablets, but liquid colourants used for cake icing are equally effective.

TECHNIQUE:

- A protective bib is placed over the patient so that their clothing is not inadvertently marked
- The patient is given one disclosing tablet and asked to chew it for about 1 min
- After this time, they are asked to spit out the chewed tablet and saliva, but are instructed not to rinse their mouth out
- Using a patient mirror, any stained plaque is pointed out by the oral health team, and the worst areas are noted (very often the gingival margins or around uneven teeth)
- Detailed advice is then given on how to improve their toothbrushing and cleaning techniques to eliminate the plaque from these areas
- The patient can follow these instructions immediately so that all the stained plaque is removed while under the supervision of the oral health team
- This enables the patient to learn more thorough and more effective techniques for plaque removal, especially in the identified heavily stained areas
- With the plaque easily visible due to the disclosing agent, the patient is able to see their progress and develop the skill to maintain good oral hygiene

BACKGROUND INFORMATION OF PROCEDURE – TOOTHBRUSHING

Toothbrushing is the most commonly used method by patients to remove plaque from the easily accessible flat surfaces of the teeth, but not from the interdental areas unless a sonic-type electric brush is used (Figure 2.4).

Many toothbrushing techniques have been suggested over the years – especially side-to-side brushing and rotary brushing – but the technique used is immaterial as long as the plaque is removed successfully without causing damage to the tooth surface. Disclosing agents can be used to determine the most successful method for a patient.

When performed thoroughly and to a consistently high standard, manual brushing with a good quality brush should be just as effective as that completed with a good quality electric brush on the flat surfaces of the teeth, but the latter takes the effort out of good brushing for those patients who lack the time and skill to perform manual brushing well.

When toothbrushing is combined with the application of a fluoridated toothpaste, the teeth and gums are cleaned free of plaque, and the teeth are protected from dental caries by the action of fluoride on the tooth enamel.

ORAL HYGIENE INSTRUCTION

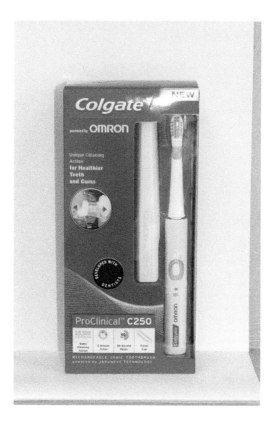

Figure 2.4 Example of sonic-style electric toothbrush

DETAILS OF PROCEDURE – TOOTHBRUSHING

Good toothbrushing aims to remove plaque from the gingival margins and some stagnation areas of the teeth and to protect the tooth surface from carious attack with a layer of fluoride.

Many toothpastes are available (fluoridated, tartar controlling, desensitising, whitening, etc.; Figure 2.5), and the oral health team will advise on the most suitable to be used in each case – patients who have no gum disease issues; for example, do not need to use toothpaste specifically to treat gum disease, and so on.

Similarly, many toothbrush designs are available – both manual and electric – but as a general rule, the head should be small to allow easier manoeuvrability, and the bristles should be multi-tufted and made of medium nylon. Even so, some patients brush with such force that they actually 'saw' into the necks of their teeth and produce abrasion cavities (Figure 2.6).

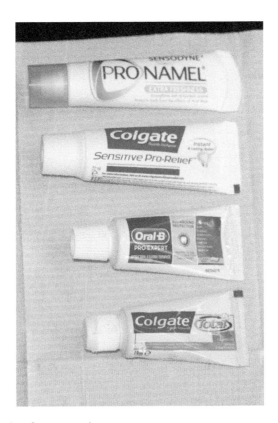

Figure 2.5 Examples of various toothpastes

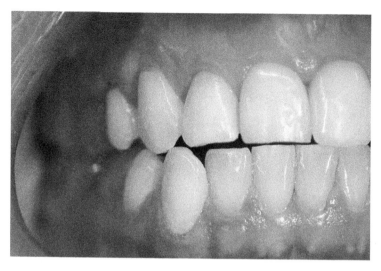

Figure 2.6 Abrasion cavity at the neck of a canine tooth caused by heavy-handed toothbrushing

ORAL HYGIENE INSTRUCTION

TECHNIQUE:

- Identify those patients with regular residual plaque after toothbrushing
- Apply a small amount of toothpaste to the patient's brush, then allow them to brush their teeth in their usual way and at their usual speed
- Disclose the residual plaque once they have finished brushing to identify the areas of its continued accumulation
- Develop a more thorough brushing technique with the patient to remove all the plaque, particularly that which has accumulated at the gingival margins (Figure 2.7)
- This may involve a change of brush from manual to electric or vice versa, as well as a change of brushing technique by the patient
- Once an effective technique has been identified, a methodical approach is to be developed so that a routine brushing technique is carried out every day
- This tends to be more effective if the more difficult areas are tackled first, such as the lingual surfaces of the lower teeth
- The patient then systematically brushes all the teeth, starting in the same place and ending in the same place each time
- Advice can then be given on the frequency of brushing – usually twice daily as a minimum, but some patients may continue with a high-sugar diet and need to brush after each meal
- Full dietary advice should also be discussed and ideally adjusted where necessary, especially for those patients identified as having a high sugar or dietary acid intake
- Toothbrushes should be replaced once the bristles start to splay, as they will not remove plaque effectively when worn down (Figure 2.8)

ORAL HYGIENE INSTRUCTION

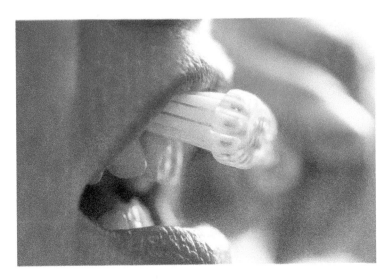

Figure 2.7 Toothbrushing the gingival margins

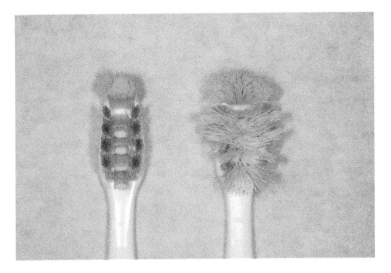

Figure 2.8 Comparison of new and worn toothbrush

BACKGROUND INFORMATION OF PROCEDURE – INTERDENTAL CLEANING

The surfaces of the teeth that remain untouched by routine toothbrushing are the contact points or interdental areas – the points where the 'front' (mesial surface) of one tooth touches the 'back' (distal surface) of the adjacent tooth in each quadrant of the dentition (Figure 2.9). Plaque accumulates here just as easily as on the flat surfaces of the teeth, and

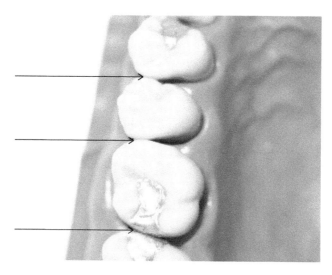

Figure 2.9 Contact points of the teeth (arrowed)

even more so when restorations extend into the interdental areas, as microscopically, the restoration margins provide a greater surface area for plaque to accumulate.

Although toothbrushes are too large to clean interdentally, other oral health products have been designed to do so:

- Tape or floss – ideal for dislodging food debris that is trapped at the contact point itself
- Manual interdental brushes – ideal for physically cleaning the interdental area (the mesial and distal surfaces of the adjacent teeth)
- Dental wood sticks – not usually recommended for use by the oral health team, as they can splinter during use or exert excessive force on the soft tissues, as can plastic alternatives
- Some specialised electric toothbrush heads
- Some mouthwashes
- Waterpik devices

The first four are used to physically clean plaque and food debris from the interdental areas, while some mouthwashes can be vigorously rinsed and swished through the interdental areas by the patient to dislodge larger particles of debris. Alternatively, a water pick device can be used to achieve the same aim.

The patient requires a certain amount of manual dexterity to use dental tape or floss effectively, and a lack of dexterity is often the cause of patients abandoning the technique. Some products have been developed to help, whereby a fork design holds a small piece of tape or floss firmly while it is used with one hand to enter and clean the interdental areas – often referred to as 'flossettes' (Figure 2.10). This removes the need for the patient to wrap the tape around the fingers and hold it firmly while trying to access the interdental areas.

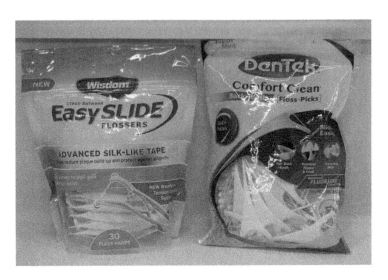

Figure 2.10 Interdental 'flossettes'

DETAILS OF PROCEDURE – FLOSSING

This is the technique used by many patients who routinely clean interdentally despite it being the most difficult to achieve.

Some tapes and flosses are waxed to assist easier entry through tight contact points, and others are impregnated with fluoride so that the interdental surfaces of the teeth are protected from tooth decay once accessed (Figure 2.11).

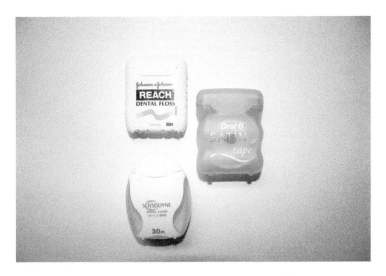

Figure 2.11 Examples of dental floss and tape products

TECHNIQUE:

- Ideally, the patient should carry out flossing with the aid of a mirror in a well-lit room
- A piece of tape or floss (approximately 20 cm) is removed from the holder and wrapped around both index fingers, leaving a central portion between the hands (Figure 2.12)
- This is held over both thumb pads and guided into each interdental area, one at a time
- Once in the area, the thumbs are used to adapt the tape to first the surface of one tooth and then the other, forming the contact point (Figure 2.13)
- While in contact with the tooth surface, the tape is drawn from side to side to wipe any plaque from each surface
- As the tape is dirtied, it is loaded off one finger and onto the other so that a clean portion is available for the next interdental area
- Tape is gentler on the gingivae than floss if the patient is heavy-handed or if force is required to access some tight interdental areas, but some patients may find tape too thick to use effectively

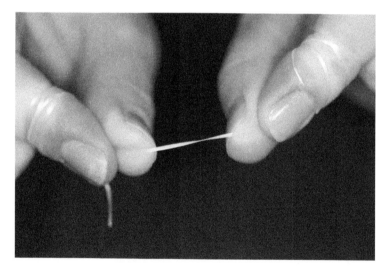

Figure 2.12 Correct positioning of floss around fingers

DETAILS OF PROCEDURE – INTERDENTAL BRUSHING

This is an alternative and useful technique for cleaning the interdental areas of patients who have contact points wide enough to admit a specially designed interdental brush into the area. Several 'bottle-brush' style designs of interdental brush are available, and a selection of popular examples is shown in Figure 2.14. These brushes are provided in a

ORAL HYGIENE INSTRUCTION

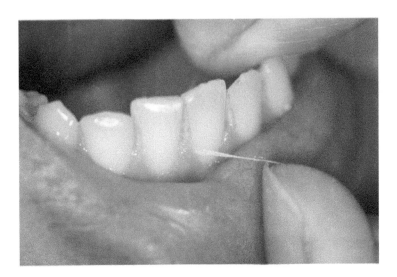

Figure 2.13 Flossing technique

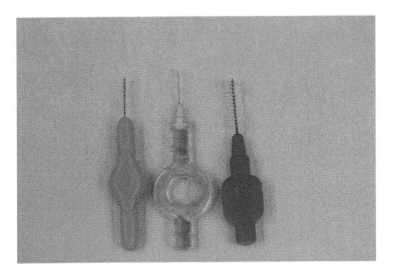

Figure 2.14 Selection of popular interdental brushes

variety of colour-coded width sizes so that patients with spaced teeth can successfully use larger brushes to clean their interdental areas, while patients with tight contact points are also able to insert the smallest design of brush to clean their interdental areas and then replace the colour-coded size when necessary (Figure 2.15).

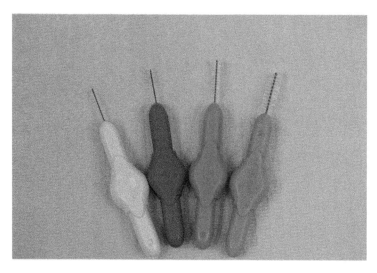

Figure 2.15 Colour-coded size examples of one interdental brush design

TECHNIQUE:

- Ideally, the patient should carry out interdental brushing with the aid of a mirror in a well-lit room
- The oral health team should advise the patient on the correct size of interdental brush to use
- Some patients may require to use more than one size of brush for different areas of their mouth, while other patients may need to use only one size of interdental brush for cleaning one specific area of their mouth
- Depending on the area of the mouth to be cleaned, the brush head can be angled to make its insertion into the interdental area easier to achieve – this is particularly useful when cleaning between posterior teeth (Figure 2.16)
- Ideally, the patient should be encouraged to place a smear of toothpaste onto the brush head before its insertion into each interdental area – the cleaning chemicals and fluoride in the toothpaste are then best placed to optimise the patient's cleaning efforts
- The brush head is pushed into the interdental area, then used in a backwards and forward motion to clean plaque from each side of the adjacent teeth and to dislodge any food debris present
- The brush can also be rotated while inserted in the interdental area to give better tooth contact and debris removal
- Any visible debris on the brush bristles must be removed by rinsing before the next contact point is accessed; otherwise, plaque and food debris will be transferred from one area to another
- Dislodged food particles in the mouth can be spat into the sink or swallowed
- The interdental brush can be rinsed clean and re-used until it becomes ineffective at cleaning or the bristles become bent, at which point it should be replaced

ORAL HYGIENE INSTRUCTION

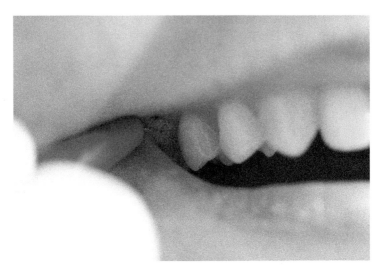

Figure 2.16 Use of interdental brush for posterior cleaning

Some good-quality electric toothbrushes have specifically designed interdental cleaning attachments that can be used by the patient in a similar way to the manual ones to ensure that plaque and food debris are removed from the contact points (Figure 2.17).

Again, the interdental area must be wide enough to allow their safe use, and the patient should follow the manufacturer's instructions or, ideally be instructed by the oral health team on their correct use.

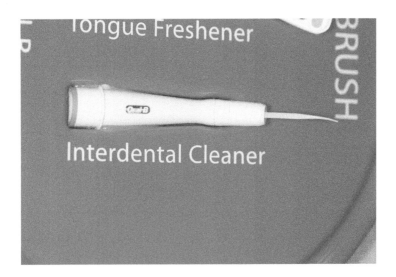

Figure 2.17 Electric brush attachment for interdental cleaning

BACKGROUND OF PROCEDURE – DIETARY ADVICE

Good dietary advice is essential in helping patients to reduce their intake, or ideally to avoid, those types of foods and drinks that are especially damaging to the teeth – those containing free sugars and those that are acidic. If patients choose to include these types of foods and drinks in their diet, they should be persuaded to confine them to their main mealtimes and then carry out some form of oral hygiene after each meal to limit the tooth damage potential the products pose. So particularly, patients should be educated in the art of 'healthy snacking' – to have safer alternatives of foods and drinks between meals which are less likely to cause tooth decay, as it is often difficult for everyone to be continually cleaning their teeth after every food or drink intake throughout the day. In essence, then, the dental team needs to provide the necessary information for the patients to understand the relevant issues of snacking between meals so that they can modify their diet accordingly.

DETAILS OF PROCEDURE – DIETARY ADVICE

The dental teams must be realistic in the dietary advice they give to patients if they are to accept and follow that advice – expecting them to cut out all forms of free sugars and acids is completely unrealistic. Rather, the dental team should focus their advice on the following:

- Introducing the patients to 'hidden sugars' in foods – where free sugars (those that can cause dental caries) have been artificially added to improve taste or for preservation purposes (Figure 2.18)
- To confine these products to mealtimes only wherever possible and then carry out some form of oral hygiene after the meal, even if that involves just using sugar-free chewing gum for 10 min

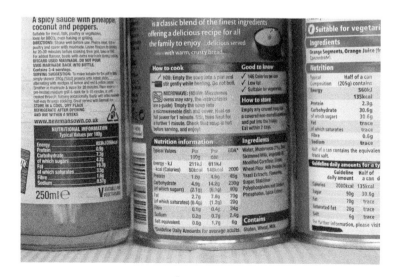

Figure 2.18 Examples of hidden sugar foods (savoury marinade, soup and tinned oranges)

ORAL HYGIENE INSTRUCTION

- Informing the patients of examples of foods and drinks containing hidden sugars so they are more aware of the issue, including the following products:
  - Cooking sauces, especially those with a tomato base
  - Table sauces, including ketchup, mayonnaise and some salad dressings
  - Flavoured crisps, such as prawn cocktail and smokey bacon.
  - Fruits tinned in syrup
  - Some tinned vegetables, including baked beans and sweetcorn
  - Many flavoured breakfast cereals
  - Jams, marmalades and chutneys
  - Some low-fat products – sugar is often artificially added to improve the taste
  - Tinned/packet soups
  - Savoury crackers and biscuits
  - Some processed ready meals
  - Energy drinks, some smoothies and flavoured yoghurts
  - Some healthy food breakfast bars
  - Dried fruits – the drying process releases the natural fruit sugars and also intensifies them
- Providing the patients with information about 'bad snacks' that should be avoided between meals – foods and drinks that contain free sugars or acids that will cause a degree of tooth decay if taken regularly:
  - Sweets and other confectionery
  - Biscuits, cakes and sweet pastries
  - Carbonated (fizzy) drinks, including 'zero sugar' products – the fizziness is still damaging to the teeth as it is acidic
  - Pure citrus fruit juices – the juicing process releases the acids and natural sugars of the fruit in a state that can affect the teeth
  - Tea and coffee with sugar
- Providing the patients with information about 'good snacks' – foods and drinks that can be safely consumed between mealtimes that will have the least likelihood of damaging their teeth:
  - Milk, ideally skimmed or semi-skimmed rather than full-fat
  - Tea and coffee with sweeteners rather than sugar
  - Non-carbonated flavoured water drinks with sweetener rather than sugar
  - Non-citrus fruits such as apples, pears and peaches
  - Fibrous raw vegetables such as carrots and celery
  - Unflavoured crisps (so simple 'ready salted' or 'cheese and onion' flavours)
  - Low-fat cheese
  - Unsweetened yoghurt

For those patients who engage with the dental team and are keen to be advised, they should be encouraged to check the product labels when they shop so that hidden sugars are identified in the foods and drinks they normally buy. Super-keen patients should be encouraged to 'grow their own' fruit and vegetables if they have space (and that required is considerably less than many assume), and ultimately become involved in cooking their own products rather than relying on unhealthy processed foods in their diet.

Finally, many foods and drinks that are linked with dental caries often tend to be linked to unwanted weight gain and obesity issues, so advice from the dental team on these topics should help some patients achieve improvements in their general health too.

Chapter 3

Scaling and polishing

REASON FOR PROCEDURE

Everyone's mouth contains a variety of bacteria, some of which react with saliva and the food eaten to produce a sticky film called plaque. Plaque forms wherever the food debris becomes lodged in the mouth, the usual areas being along the gum margin (see Figure 2.3) and in difficult-to-clean areas called stagnation areas. Examples include the interdental areas of the teeth and around the margins of restorations.

Plaque lying along the gum margin will irritate the soft tissues and eventually cause inflammation of the gums or gingivitis. Regular toothbrushing and interdental cleaning by the patient will remove the plaque and prevent this from happening.

However, if the plaque is not removed, it gradually hardens by absorbing minerals from the patient's saliva and becomes calculus (tartar). Calculus cannot be removed by toothbrushing alone, and the dentist, therapist or hygienist will need to remove it by scaling the teeth. When the plaque or calculus is attached to the tooth surface above the gum line, it is called 'supragingival' (Figure 3.1).

If the calculus is left untouched, it gradually forms further and further down the side of the tooth root as the gum tissue is destroyed. Eventually, the tooth's supporting structures (the jawbone and periodontal ligaments) are also destroyed. The tooth becomes loose in its socket. This is called periodontal disease, or periodontitis; the plaque and calculus present beneath the gum is referred to as 'subgingival'.

The more advanced the damage to the periodontal tissues, the more difficult it is for the oral health team to treat, and the more likely that long-term problems including tooth loss will occur.

The procedures discussed are:

- Simple scaling of supragingival debris
- Deep scaling and root surface debridement of subgingival debris
- Use of periodontal adjuncts
- Polishing and air abrasion for stain removal

Basic Guide to Dental Procedures, Third Edition. Carole Hollins.
© 2024 John Wiley & Sons Ltd. Published 2024 by John Wiley & Sons Ltd.

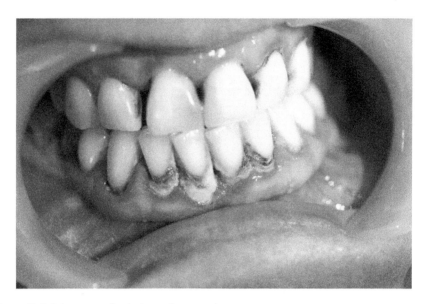

Figure 3.1 Supragingival calculus on lower teeth

BACKGROUND INFORMATION OF PROCEDURE – SCALING

The dentist, therapist or hygienist can scale a patient's teeth using hand instruments, electrical scalers or a combination of both. The procedure aims to remove all the calculus and plaque from around each tooth so that the supporting structures are no longer irritated and inflamed and can repair themselves.

If the calculus has extended down the side of the root and under the gum (subgingival), its removal is more difficult to achieve. Electric scalers vibrate ultrasonically and have a spray of water at their tip to help remove the calculus both from the tooth root and out from under the gum (Figure 3.2).

Some patients find the vibration and cold water uncomfortable and may choose to have a scaling procedure carried out under local anaesthetic.

DETAILS OF PROCEDURE – SIMPLE SCALING

The presence of supragingival plaque and calculus will have been noticed by the dentist during a routine examination of the patient's mouth or been discovered lying interdentally after radiographs have been taken (Figure 3.3). The amount present and whether local anaesthesia is required will help determine whether a second appointment will be needed or if the scaling can be completed during the examination appointment. The dentist, therapist or hygienist will act as the operator to carry out the procedure while assisted by the dental nurse.

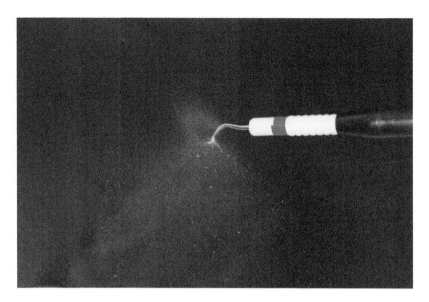

Figure 3.2 Ultrasonic scaler showing water spray effect

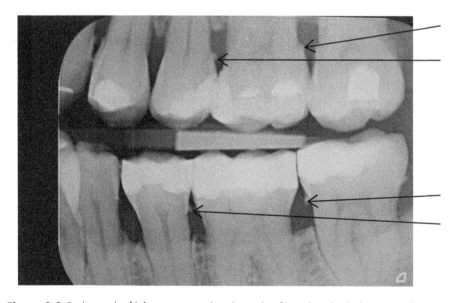

Figure 3.3 Radiograph of left posterior teeth with specks of interdental calculus arrowed

Supragingival scaling removes plaque and calculus deposits from the enamel surface of the teeth down to the gingival margins of the teeth. The hand instruments used are shaped accordingly to fit around the shape of the teeth (sickle and Jaquette scalers) or are shaped like a fine chisel (push scaler) to be pushed between the anterior teeth to remove interdental calculus (Figure 3.4).

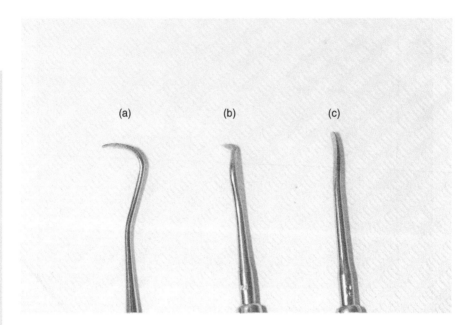

Figure 3.4 Supragingival scalers. (a) Sickle scaler. (b) Jaquette scaler. (c) Push scaler

In addition, a high-speed suction tip is used by the dental nurse to suck up water and dislodged debris from the patient's mouth during the procedure, while tissues or gauze sheets are used to periodically wipe the debris from the instruments.

The instruments and materials that may be required to carry out a simple scale and polish procedure are shown in Figure 3.5.

TECHNIQUE:

- The oral health team and the patient wear personal protective equipment (Figure 3.6)
- Local anaesthetic is given if required
- Hand and/or electric scalers are made ready
- If an electric scaler is used, the dental nurse uses high-speed suction to remove water and debris from the patient's mouth as the scaling is carried out
- The operator will systematically scale each tooth that has calculus present, using vision and tactile sensation to determine when it has been fully removed
- The scaler is worked from the bottom edge of the calculus upwards in a scraping motion, so that it is dislodged 'en masse'
- The instrument is then reapplied to remove any remaining specks of calculus until a smooth tooth surface is achieved (Figure 3.7)
- The process causes some amount of bleeding of the gums as they are in an inflamed state, but scaling does not cut into the gums themselves
- The gums will return to their healthy pink appearance within days of the calculus being removed

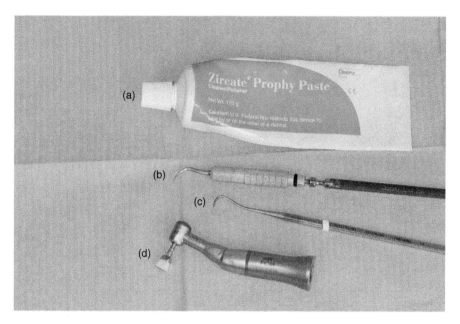

Figure 3.5 Instruments and materials for simple scale and polish procedure. (a) Prophylaxis paste. (b) Ultrasonic scaler. (c) Hand scaler. (d) Polishing brush with handpiece

DETAILS OF PROCEDURE – DEEP SCALING AND DEBRIDEMENT

The presence of subgingival plaque and calculus is determined by the dentist while carrying out a basic periodontal examination of the teeth, and the presence and depth of any periodontal pockets are recorded. Plaque retention factors such as overhanging fillings are also noted.

Deep scaling and debridement are usually carried out under local anaesthetic and in a few sections of the mouth at a time, and the number of areas to be treated determines the number of appointments required. Subgingival scaling removes plaque and calculus deposits from the root surfaces of teeth within the periodontal pockets. In addition, the instruments are also used to remove a layer of contaminated cementum from the root surfaces during debridement, and the debris created is then irrigated from the pockets and aspirated from the mouth.

The instruments used to achieve subgingival scaling and debridement must be long enough to reach the base of each periodontal pocket and thin enough to do so without tearing the soft tissues – they are called curettes (Figure 3.8). The ultrasonic scaler unit has interchangeable heads to be used for both supragingival and subgingival scaling and debridement procedures.

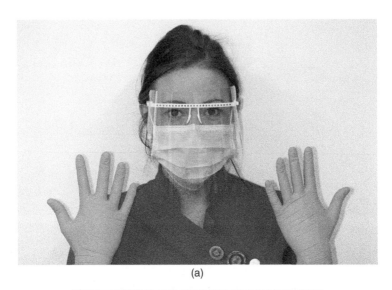

(a)

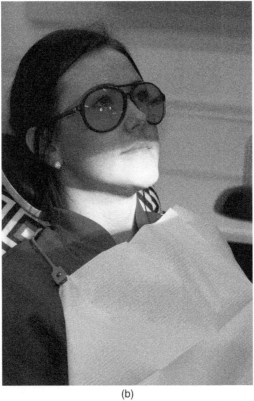

(b)

Figure 3.6 Personal protective equipment. (a) Oral health team members – gloves, mask and eye protection. (b) Patient – waterproof bib and safety glasses

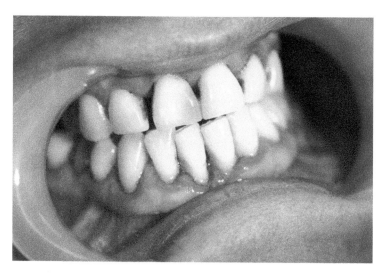

Figure 3.7 Appearance after completion of supragingival scaling

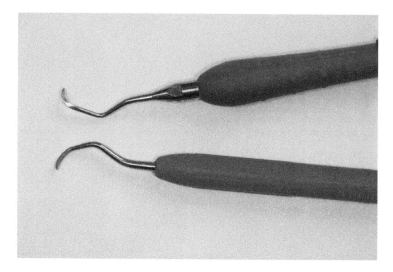

Figure 3.8 Curettes for subgingival scaling and debridement

TECHNIQUE:

- The oral health team and the patient wear personal protective equipment
- Local anaesthetic is administered as required; the particular equipment and materials that may be required to do so are shown in Figure 3.9

(continued)

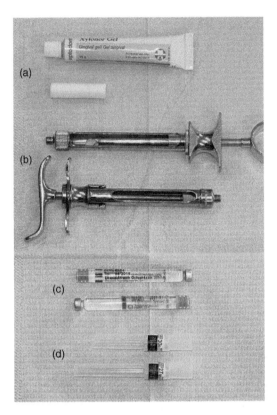

Figure 3.9 Local anaesthetic equipment. (a) Topical anaesthetic and cotton wool roll. (b) Syringe – aspirating or non-aspirating. (c) Cartridge – content specific to patient needs. (d) Needle – long or short

TECHNIQUE: (*Continued*)

- Curettes and the ultrasonic unit are ready
- The dental nurse uses high-speed suction to remove water and debris from the patient's mouth as the scaling and debridement procedures are carried out
- The operator will systematically deep scale each root in the anaesthetised mouth section that has calculus present, using vision and tactile sensation to determine when it has been fully removed
- The curette is worked from the bottom edge of the calculus upwards in a scraping motion, so that it is dislodged 'en masse'
- The instrument will then be reapplied to remove a layer of contaminated cementum from the root surface during debridement, the process being repeated until a smooth root surface is achieved
- Deep pockets may be irrigated with antiseptic mouthwash solutions by some operators to assist in the destruction and removal of the periodontal bacteria

DETAILS OF PROCEDURE – USE OF PERIODONTAL ADJUNCTS

While periodontal disease develops over time in patients with consistently poor oral hygiene, there are several known risk factors that allow the condition to persist or even worsen despite the best efforts of the well-motivated patient. In these cases, the dental team may use periodontal adjuncts to assist in managing the disease and help to bring localized areas of infection under control. By definition, adjuncts are auxiliary treatments used on a temporary basis to help improve the overall condition and produce a period of stability in the disease process.

Several products are available for use, but they are all used in a similar fashion – the patient undergoes a thorough deep scaling and debridement of the affected areas as described previously. Then, the chosen adjunct is placed into the cleaned 'pockets' of the gums in the problem areas. The adjuncts contain chemicals that act against the bacteria involved in periodontal disease by killing them, often by a slow-release action with chemicals such as chlorhexidine (which is found in some toothpastes and mouthwashes), while others contain antibiotics that are particularly effective against the types of bacteria found in the periodontal pockets. Examples of gel-type products are shown in Figure 3.10a, while a type of slow-release adjunct is shown in Figure 3.10b. This latter product has the adjunct held on a plastic-like 'chip' that is pushed under the gum and into the pocket, where it remains for up to 3 months while slowly releasing the bactericidal chemical directly in the area of bacterial contamination.

BACKGROUND INFORMATION OF PROCEDURE – POLISHING AND AIR ABRASION

Whether calculus is present or not, everyone's teeth can stain from time to time by exposure to normal dietary substances such as tea, coffee, red wine and highly coloured foods. Smokers can also develop unsightly dark staining from tobacco tar products.

The process of professional polishing of the anterior teeth using special abrasive pastes can easily remove all but the most tenacious of these surface stains, giving the teeth a cleaner and brighter appearance. Similarly, the process of stain removal using an air abrasion attachment to the dental handpiece and special abrasive powders is equally effective and is particularly useful in removing tenacious tar stains.

Obviously, continued exposure to the staining agents will cause the discolouration to develop again with time, but it can usually be kept under control if the patient has a good and regular oral hygiene routine. In particular, the regular use of 'whitening' toothpastes or mouthwashes may help in some cases to keep tooth surface staining to a minimum. However, patients must realise that despite being marketed as 'whitening' products, these toothpastes and mouthwashes do not change the actual colour of the teeth (they do not 'whiten' the teeth) but act simply by removing surface stains. So, if a patient has naturally yellow, grey or cream-coloured teeth, their tooth colour will remain unchanged no matter how frequently these products are used. Some 'whitening' products available act by chemically reacting with the surface stains to remove them, while others contain microcrystals or other abrasives to physically scour the tooth surface and remove the stains. Overusing the more abrasive products should be discouraged as the tooth enamel may become damaged in some cases. Professional polishing and air abrasion cause no surface damage to the teeth. Professional tooth whitening procedures and products are discussed in Chapter 13.

SCALING AND POLISHING

SCALING AND POLISHING

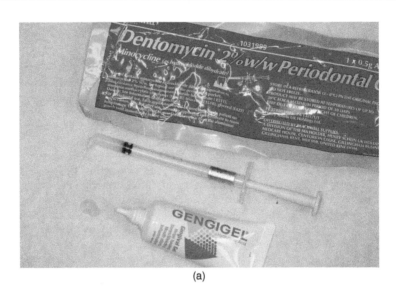

(a)

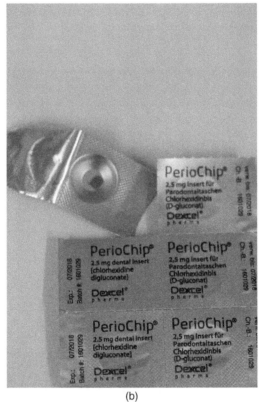

(b)

Figure 3.10 Examples of periodontal adjuncts. (a) Periodontal subgingival gel examples. (b) 'Periochips'

DETAILS OF PROCEDURE – POLISHING AND AIR ABRASION

Polishing is usually carried out at the end of a course of treatment, especially once scaling has been completed. The use of bristle brushes or rubber cups in the dental handpiece (Figure 3.11) to apply the abrasive polishing paste gives a greater cleaning effect than if it were applied using a toothbrush. The pastes are often flavoured for the benefit of the patient and feel quite gritty in the mouth.

Air abrasion is often carried out just as necessary rather than at the end of a course of treatment, as it tends to be used specifically for the removal of tenacious stains that build up on a regular basis – such as tar staining seen in smokers. A specialised attachment is connected to the dental handpiece adaptor so that compressed air is available to deliver the abrasion powder (Figure 3.12). Again, the powders are flavoured for the benefit of the patient.

TECHNIQUES:

- If not already in place, the operator, nurse and patient wear personal protective equipment
- Either a bristle brush or rubber cup will be locked into the dental handpiece and then dabbed into the polishing paste so that a small amount is picked up
- With the lips held out of the way, the rotating brush/cup will be moved across the front surface of each anterior tooth, from one contact point to the next, until the stains are removed
- The patient may feel a not unpleasant tickling sensation in each tooth

(continued)

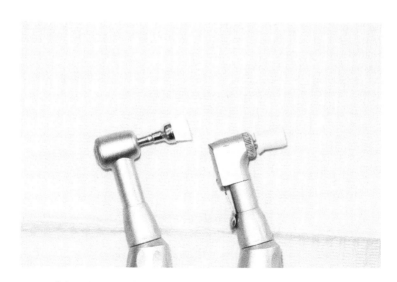

Figure 3.11 Polishing brush and cup in dental handpieces

SCALING AND POLISHING

SCALING AND POLISHING

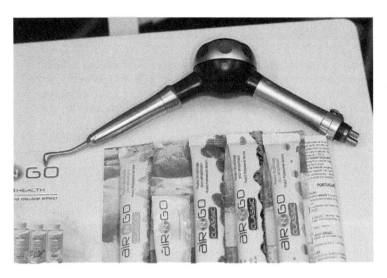

Figure 3.12 Air abrasion head and selection of flavoured abrasion powders

TECHNIQUE: (*Continued*)

- The brush will be worked over the whole tooth surface, especially into the contact points of the teeth, where stains usually accumulate
- Fresh paste is picked up on the brush for each tooth
- Once the procedure is complete, the patient can rinse the gritty paste out of the mouth
- With the air abrasion technique, the gritty powders are blasted onto the tooth surfaces to be cleaned by the use of compressed air from the dental handpiece adaptor
- While the abrasion head can be angled to direct the powder jet onto the teeth, there is likely to be a degree of spatter onto the soft tissues, and this can cause mild irritation of these tissues in some cases
- Consequently, it is usual to smear the soft tissues around the teeth with petroleum jelly before proceeding with air abrasion, and the dental nurse will also use high-speed suction to remove as much spatter as possible during the procedure

Chapter 4

Diagnostic techniques

When a patient attends a dental appointment for a dental examination, the dentist has to check the oral health and determine the presence and location of caries, periodontal disease or oral soft tissue problems. While the dentist's visual skills are paramount in identifying problems of the oral tissues, it is often necessary for diagnostic techniques to be implemented so that a definitive diagnosis can be made.

The four techniques discussed are:

- Visual skills
- Use of dental hand instruments
- Dental radiographs – conventional, digital and cone-beam computer tomography (CBCT)
- Study models

BACKGROUND INFORMATION OF PROCEDURE – VISUAL SKILLS

When patients attend a dental examination, many believe that the dentist checks their teeth and gums for signs of tooth decay or gum disease, notes how well or not their tooth brushing is and treats any dental problems that have been noticed. In reality, the dentist uses their visual skills as soon as the patient enters the surgery – checking the general appearance of the patient, whether they look well or not, whether they appear anxious or fearful, whether they seem happy and comfortable or upset, and so on. Any issues noticed at this point can then be checked and discussed with the patient before the actual dental examination begins.

Most dentists carry out a dental examination methodically so as not to miss any areas to be checked, often using written or computer templates as prompts to remind them to check certain points as they proceed through the examination process. This will include checking and updating the patient's medical history before discussing any specific issues

Basic Guide to Dental Procedures, Third Edition. Carole Hollins.
© 2024 John Wiley & Sons Ltd. Published 2024 by John Wiley & Sons Ltd.

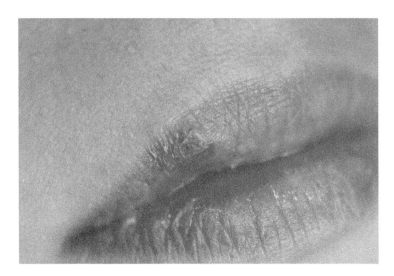

Figure 4.1 'Cold sore' lesion on the upper lip

of concern, either medical or dental. Many then check the patient's extra-oral (outside the mouth) appearance first, whether all looks well or whether abnormalities are noted, such as swellings, skin discolouration, lesions present and so on (Figure 4.1).

The examination then progresses to checking the intra-oral (inside the mouth) structures, including the soft tissues within the oral cavity, such as the cheeks, the roof of the mouth, the tongue and the tonsils at the back of the mouth. Most dentists will use a small mouth mirror to assist them at this point, as the mirror has multiple functions – it can be angled to view difficult-to-see areas and structures at the back of the mouth, with or without light reflection, as well as to retract soft tissues such as the lips, cheeks or tongue so that other structures can be seen more clearly. Any soft tissue findings may seem innocuous to the patient, but to the dental team, they provide lots of information. They may even lead to diagnoses of diseases or disorders that need further treatment. For example, Figure 4.2 shows the classic appearance of cheek biting, indicating the patient may also clench and grind their teeth and may become prone to tooth fractures in the future. Figure 4.3 shows a recurrent ulcer on the inside of the lower lip, which sometimes indicates the patient has a nutritional deficiency. Figure 4.4 shows a lesion on the right border of the tongue that may be due to trauma but could also be an early cancerous lesion that requires urgent referral and treatment. Figure 4.5 shows the typical appearance of an inflamed palate (roof of the mouth) in a long-standing smoker – a condition called 'stomatitis nicotina' that requires regular checking and monitoring in case of any sinister change. Finally, Figure 4.6 shows a swollen left tonsil and the presence of several white 'tonsilar stones' within the structure of the tonsil surface, indicating the patient has, or has recently had, a viral throat infection. All these examples were incidental findings during routine dental examinations undertaken by the author over several years, but the importance of using adequate visual skills cannot be overemphasised, as the patient with the tongue lesion did indeed have an early oral cancer development.

Once the dentist has completed the soft tissue examinations, they will progress to checking the hard tissues – the teeth. Before beginning to check for dental caries, though,

DIAGNOSTIC TECHNIQUES

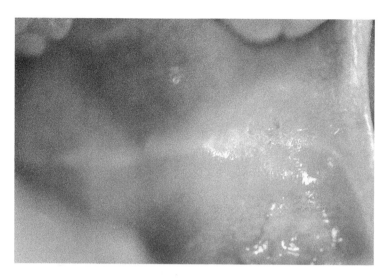

Figure 4.2 Cheek ridge indicating possible clenching and grinding habits

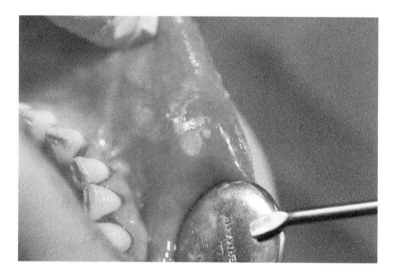

Figure 4.3 Recurrent ulcer inside the lower lip

the dentist will visually inspect the teeth for any signs of tooth wear due to causes other than decay, as these causes are equally likely to result in the patient requiring tooth restoration or even extraction if they remain undiagnosed. The three most common causes of tooth surface loss besides dental caries are abrasion (Figure 4.7), attrition (Figure 4.8a and b) and erosion (Figure 4.9a and b).

Abrasion affects the flat surfaces of the teeth against the lips and cheeks. It is usually caused by heavy-handed toothbrushing, where the patient uses a backwards and forwards 'sawing' action of brushing that wears into the necks of the teeth and results in

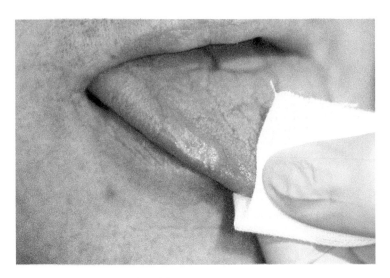

Figure 4.4 Lesion on the right border of the tongue

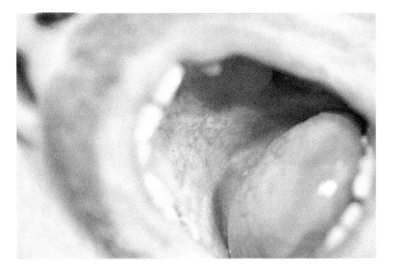

Figure 4.5 Typical appearance of 'stomatitis nicotina' on the roof of the mouth in a smoker

sensitivity or pain. Once diagnosed, the patient is instructed in correct brushing techniques to prevent further damage and the affected teeth can then be restored.

Attrition affects the biting surfaces of the teeth and is usually caused by the patient subconsciously clenching and grinding their teeth over a period of time, often while concentrating or carrying out repetitive tasks, and especially while asleep. The constant grinding action wears the biting edges of the front teeth down so that they chip and splinter away, while the back teeth develop enamel cracks or even fracture off pieces of the tooth. Once diagnosed, the patient is counselled and often fitted with a guard to wear

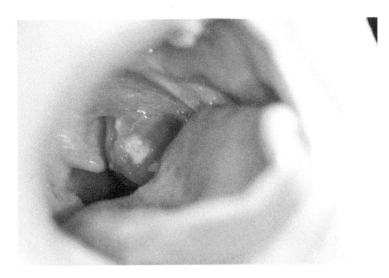

Figure 4.6 Swollen left tonsil with 'stones' present

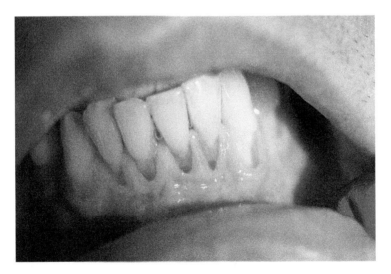

Figure 4.7 Abrasion damage affecting the lower anterior teeth

(especially when the grinding occurs during sleep) so that the damage is limited and the affected teeth can be restored.

Erosion can affect either the flat surface of the front teeth or the biting surface of the back teeth and is usually caused by the intake of excessive amounts of dietary acids, especially in liquid forms such as fizzy drinks, sports drinks, fruit juices and alcohol such as wines and fizzy or fruity mixers. However, in some patients, erosion can also be caused by digestive problems that result in acid reflux or with psychological conditions resulting

DIAGNOSTIC TECHNIQUES

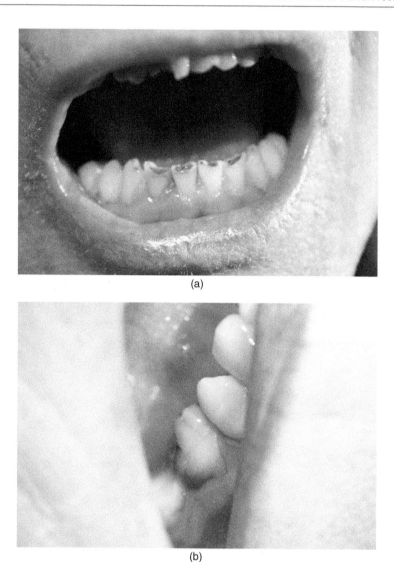

(a)

(b)

Figure 4.8 Attrition damage. (a) Edge wear of lower anterior teeth. (b) Wear crack of a lower molar tooth

in repeated vomiting, such as bulimia. Where dietary acids are not the cause of the erosion, the affected patients require medical intervention as well as dental treatment.

Where dietary acids are involved, the tooth enamel is gradually eroded so the underlying yellow dentine is exposed and the teeth become sensitive. The upper front teeth can especially wear on the surface against the lips when patients repeatedly drink directly from bottles or cans or on the surface against the roof of the mouth when acidic drinks are consumed regularly throughout the day. The back teeth erode on the biting surfaces so that enamel pits appear, and any fillings present stand higher than the tooth surface as

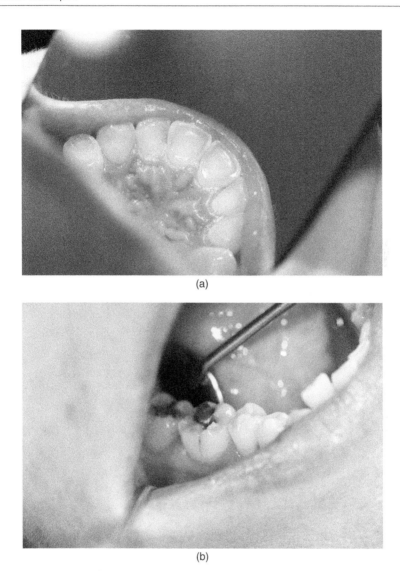

(a)

(b)

Figure 4.9 Erosion damage. (a) Palatal surface of the upper front teeth eroded down to the dentine. (b) Occlusal surface of a lower molar tooth with enamel pits and filling standing proud of tooth surface

the acids do not wear them away. Once diagnosed, the patient is advised on their dietary acid intake and how to reduce the damage occurring by confining the acids to mealtimes only and using specific oral health products that assist in enamel repair. The affected teeth are then restored.

The dental examination will then proceed to check the teeth for signs of dental caries, check the gingivae for signs of health or disease and record the occlusion where necessary using the other three techniques listed.

BACKGROUND INFORMATION OF PROCEDURE – INSTRUMENTS

A variety of dental hand instruments called probes have been designed to aid the dentist in detecting the presence of both caries and periodontal disease.

Those used to detect caries have sharp points that can be run over the tooth surface to find any softened areas of the enamel, which indicates that demineralisation has occurred and the area has undergone a carious attack.

Those used to detect periodontal disease are blunt-ended and have graded depth markings so the gums are not pierced during use, and any gum pockets discovered can be depth recorded.

DETAILS OF PROCEDURE – INSTRUMENTS

Frank carious cavities in teeth are easily visible to the dentist when they occur on uncovered and easily accessible surfaces of those teeth (Figure 4.10), but more difficult areas to examine require the use of dental probes. All have been designed so that their pointed ends are bent at various angles so that the dentist can easily probe all surfaces of each tooth (Figure 4.11).

TECHNIQUE:

- The patient is placed in the dental chair at a suitable angle for the dentist, with the dental inspection light providing good illumination when the mouth is open
- Visual examination is carried out first so that any suspicious tooth surfaces are detected
- Each suspect area is then revisited, and the probe end is run over the tooth surface
- A hard, scratchy surface indicates sound enamel
- A soft, non-scratchy surface indicates the presence of dental caries
- The dentist will be able to determine the presence of either by tactile sensation through the probe to the hand
- The dental nurse will record the findings of the dental examination on a manual chart or its computer alternative, and either can be referred to at a later date to monitor the improvement or deterioration of the patient's dental condition and any treatment that has been provided by the oral health team to treat any caries found

Periodontal disease is often more difficult to detect by vision alone as the gums of some patients appear to be quite healthy and exhibit no bleeding when touched. The presence of periodontal pockets alongside the tooth roots indicates that some destruction of the supporting tissues of the tooth has occurred – and the deeper the pocket, the more severe the destruction.

The pockets are not visible to the naked eye but can be easily detected using a periodontal probe (see Figure 4.12).

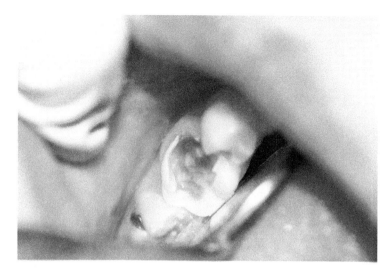

Figure 4.10 Cavity in tooth

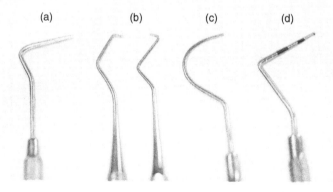

Figure 4.11 Diagnostic probes. (a) Right angle probe. (b) Briault probe (both ends). (c) Sickle probe. (d) Periodontal BPE probe

TECHNIQUE:

- The patient is placed in the dental chair at a suitable angle for the dentist, with the dental inspection light providing good illumination when the mouth is open
- Visual examination is carried out first, including the presence and location of any plaque or calculus and the identification of any tooth mobility

(continued)

DIAGNOSTIC TECHNIQUES

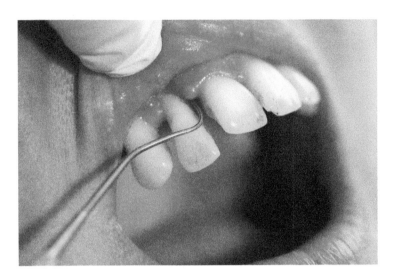

Figure 4.12 BPE probe inserted in a periodontal pocket

TECHNIQUE: (*Continued*)

- Each suspect tooth/gum junction is then inspected for periodontal pocketing by 'walking' the blunt-ended probe around the gingival crevice
- A healthy gingival crevice is no deeper than 2 mm and does not bleed when probed
- Where a periodontal problem exists, the probe sinks easily below the tooth-gum junction, and the area bleeds on probing
- The probe may sink for several millimetres, and greater depths indicate more severe periodontal disease (Figure 4.12)
- Sometimes, the probe may also detect specks of subgingival calculus on the tooth root
- The dental nurse records the findings of the periodontal examination on a manual chart or its computer alternative, and either can be referred to at a later date to monitor the improvement or deterioration of the patient's periodontal condition

BACKGROUND INFORMATION OF PROCEDURE – DENTAL RADIOGRAPHS

Radiographs allow the dentist to see within the dental tissues themselves without having to drill or cut into those tissues beforehand.

They are an invaluable diagnostic technique for determining the presence or absence of dental disease, as well as such widely varied features as unerupted teeth, jaw or tooth fractures, extra teeth, foreign bodies and so on.

A wide variety of images can be produced depending on the type of radiographic view required, ranging from a single tooth to the whole oral cavity. Where a single tooth or just a few teeth are to be viewed, an intra-oral radiograph is taken, which can then either be chemically processed to produce a hard copy image (conventional technique) or

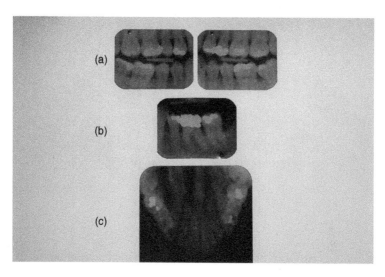

Figure 4.13 Examples of intra-oral radiographic views. (a) Bitewings (right and left). (b) Periapical. (c) Upper occlusal

transmitted with specialist digital equipment directly or via a specialist scanner device, to a computer screen for immediate viewing (digital technique).

Examples of the types of intra-oral radiographs discussed are shown in Figure 4.13 and are:

- Bitewings (right or left – showing the crowns of all upper and lower posterior/back teeth on one side)
- Periapical (showing up to four adjacent teeth in full length)
- Occlusal (showing either upper or lower anterior/front teeth at full length and their surrounding bone)

When a more extensive area is to be radiographed, an extra-oral dental pantomograph (DPT) view is taken, using a cassette containing intensifying screens to reduce the X-ray exposure of the patient. The image will show all the teeth in both the upper and lower jaws, as well as the surrounding bony anatomy (Figure 4.14). Modern DPT machines are also available using digital techniques rather than conventional techniques using cassettes.

A specialist cephalometric view (side of the head and jaws) can also be taken in certain orthodontic cases, so that measurements can be made of the angulation of the teeth, jaws and skull to each other to determine the severity of the malocclusion and the likelihood of the need for orthognathic surgery to correct the jaws. The view produced is referred to as a lateral skull image (Figure 4.15).

When a patient is being considered for the replacement of one or more missing teeth with dental implants, a specialised three-dimensional (3D) image is required that allows the dentist to visualise not just the side-to-side anatomical positions of the teeth, but also the depth (thickness) of the bone in which the teeth sit. This is called cone-beam computerised tomography (CBCT) and enables the clinician to determine the exact depth and angulation that each implant must be placed at to achieve the required restorative result

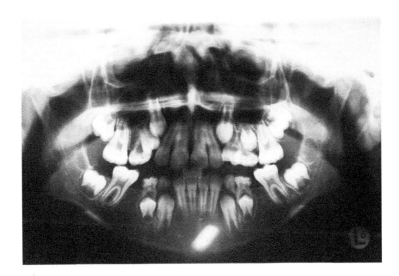

Figure 4.14 Dental pantomograph view

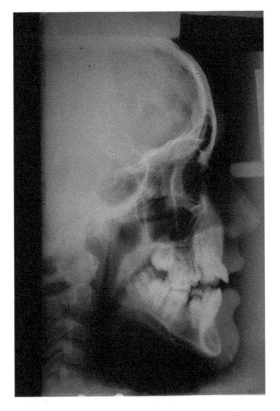

Figure 4.15 Lateral skull radiograph on viewer showing side view of the patient's skull

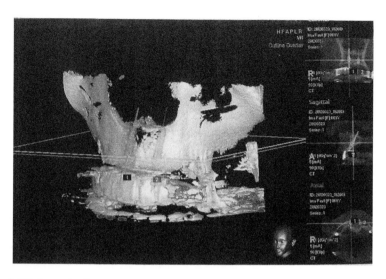

Figure 4.16 Example of a computerised 3D scan (CBCT view) for implant planning

while avoiding any damage to the surrounding anatomical structures (Figure 4.16). The technique is also used in hospitals to diagnose pathological conditions affecting the head and neck, including cancers.

DETAILS OF PROCEDURE – DENTAL RADIOGRAPHS

When an intra-oral view is taken, it is important that there is no distortion of the film or the image produced, as can happen if the film is bent in the mouth or if the angulation of the X-ray machine cone is incorrect. Therefore, the film is placed into one of a variety of holders before being positioned in the patient's mouth so that the film is held in parallel to the tooth being exposed, thereby preventing distortion as well as allowing the cone angulation to be set correctly.

If a digital radiograph is to be produced rather than a conventional one, the digital sensor/receptor unit is loaded and exposed in the same manner as the conventional film.

TECHNIQUE:

- The patient is seated comfortably in the dental chair, usually in an upright position or nearly so
- All removable prostheses are taken out of the mouth, as they superimpose their image over the teeth and make diagnosis difficult
- The X-ray machine exposure and time settings are chosen by the operator, depending on which tooth and view is being taken
- A suitable holder is chosen depending on whether a bitewing, anterior or posterior periapical view is required (Figure 4.17)

(continued)

DIAGNOSTIC TECHNIQUES

TECHNIQUE: (*Continued*)

- Occlusal views do not require the use of a holder, as the patient can bite onto the film packet itself and hold it correctly in place during exposure
- The intra-oral film is correctly inserted into the holder so that the front of the film faces the X-ray cone
- The holder and film are then gently but accurately positioned in the patient's mouth, so that the tooth to be viewed lies between the film holder and the X-ray cone, and in parallel with both (Figure 4.18)
- The final position of the X-ray cone is checked before all personnel except the patient move outside the 2 m safety zone
- The patient is told to remain completely still during the exposure, which is identified by a ringing or buzzing sound
- The operator presses the X-ray machine button to expose the film, releasing it only when the audio alarm ends
- A digital X-ray view is produced immediately on the computer screen when the sensor plate is wired directly to the computer or the receptor is scanned, and the image is then sent directly to the computer screen from the scanner (Figure 4.19)
- An ordinary (conventional) film is removed from the patient's mouth and holder, and taken to be chemically processed either manually or in an automatic processor
- The processed radiograph can be viewed on a light viewer within 5 min, and a diagnosis made
- Conventional radiographs are stored as hard copies in the patient's records, while digital radiographs are stored on the computer, although they can be printed off as hard copies if required

When a DPT or CBCT is to be taken, the patient must be correctly positioned within the headset of the X-ray machine so that the film produced is in focus throughout and that no positional distortions are produced. The machines have head positioning and jaw positioning devices incorporated into their designs to achieve this (Figure 4.20). The exposure time is longer than intra-oral views, but a reduced X-ray dose to the patient is achieved by the use of intensifying screens within the cassette on older DPT machines and digital imaging on modern DPT and CBCT machines.

The cassette film is chemically processed to produce the image, either manually or automatically for older DPT machines, or more usually with modern machines, it is sent as a digital image directly to the computer. DPT views are often taken for orthodontic diagnosis of missing or unerupted teeth, as well as to identify jaw fractures and pathology. More modern machines tend to be combinations that can take both DPT and CBCT images. The latter is particularly useful in implant cases, where a 3D image of the jaws is required to accurately position the implant from both side-to-side and forwards–backwards views.

BACKGROUND INFORMATION OF PROCEDURE – STUDY MODELS

When a patient has a complicated occlusion, it is easier for the dentist to visualise this by copying the dental arches and how they bite together by producing a set of study models

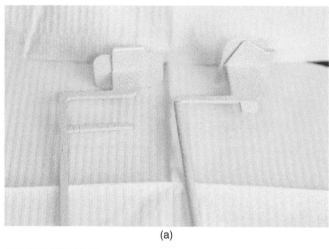

(a)

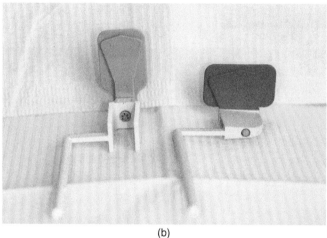

(b)

Figure 4.17 Examples of film holders. (a) Horizontal and vertical bitewing holders. (b) Anterior and posterior periapical holders.

(Figure 4.21). These can then be viewed from all angles by the dentist without the hinderance of the patient's lips, cheeks and tongue.

Often, unexpected details are discovered that were not evident just by viewing the patient in the dental chair, such as abnormal wear patterns on the teeth.

Diagnostic study models are invaluable aids to the dentist in the following situations:

- Orthodontics
- Multiple crown restorations
- Bridges
- Implants
- Bruxism (tooth grinding)
- Denture design

DIAGNOSTIC TECHNIQUES

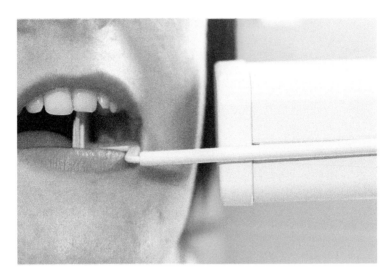

Figure 4.18 Film packet and holder in place ready for exposure

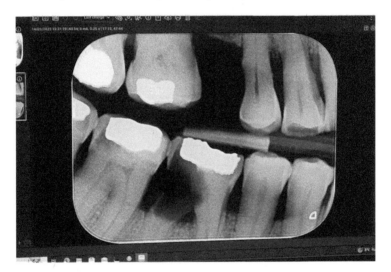

Figure 4.19 Digital image on computer screen

DETAILS OF PROCEDURE – STUDY MODELS

When producing diagnostic study models, an impression has to be taken of each arch of the patient's dentition that is accurate without being prohibitively expensive. The impression material of choice is alginate, which is sufficiently elastomeric to be accurate as well as being relatively inexpensive. Correctly sized stock trays are adequate to hold the impression material, and a wax wafer bite allows the accurate positioning of the two models produced.

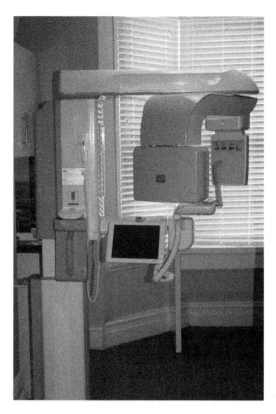

Figure 4.20 Example of a CBCT machine with handholds and head positioning features

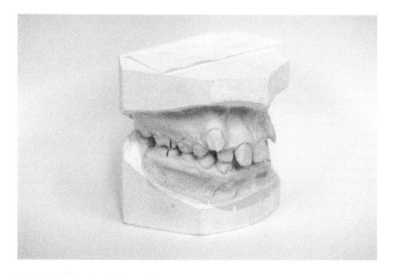

Figure 4.21 Set of simple study models

DIAGNOSTIC TECHNIQUES

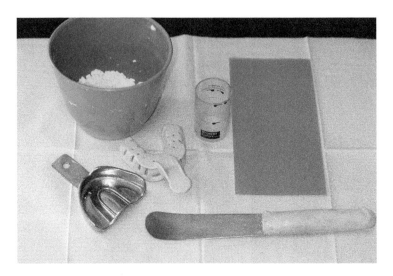

Figure 4.22 Equipment and materials for taking a set of simple study models

The materials and equipment that may be required for a set of simple study models are shown in Figure 4.22.

In more complicated cases, the models are often mounted on an articulator by the laboratory technician so that jaw movements can be reproduced and a more in-depth occlusal analysis can be carried out.

TECHNIQUE:

- The patient is usually seated upright in the dental chair so that excess material does not cause gagging during the procedure
- A protective bib is placed over the patient
- All removable prostheses are taken out of the mouth unless their presence is required for the occlusal analysis
- A wax bite is taken if necessary, using a roll of warmed pink wax placed over the lower teeth so that it is bitten into when the patient closes their jaws together, or using a material specifically designed for recording the bite that is laid over the lower teeth and bitten into until it has set by chemical reaction
- Once removed from the mouth and cooled, the now stiff wax roll or set stretch of bite material will allow the study models to be accurately positioned in the patient's bite by aligning each model into the tooth indentations recorded in the wax or bite record material
- Upper and lower stock trays are sized to the patient's dental arches, so that each arch is fully covered by the tray without being uncomfortable or choking the patient
- A stiff, bubble-free mix of alginate is prepared and loaded into one of the trays and then inserted into the patient's mouth to cover one of the dental arches fully
- The patient is advised to breathe through the nose while the impression is being taken, not to swallow, and to keep the lips and cheeks in a relaxed state

- Once set, the impression is carefully removed from the mouth in the tray and disinfected as necessary
- The process is repeated for the opposing arch
- Study models are cast in dental stone from the impressions, ideally within 24h of the impressions being taken

The technique of taking alginate impressions for study models can be carried out by suitably trained dental nurses as an extended duty, and the full procedure is discussed further in Chapter 14.

DIAGNOSTIC TECHNIQUES

Chapter 5

Tooth restoration with fillings

REASON FOR PROCEDURE

When caries attacks a tooth, a process of demineralisation occurs in the hard tissues of the tooth, starting in the enamel outer layer. This opens the inner dentine layer to infection by the bacteria involved in caries, and as this layer contains nerve endings, the patient feels hot and cold sensitivity and, eventually, pain. Once painful, there is a loss of function as the patient avoids chewing with the affected tooth.

The caries attack progresses further into the tooth until it reaches the pulp chamber, eventually causing an abscess and the death of the tooth unless the tooth is dentally treated by filling before the pulp chamber is breached.

A tooth may also require a filling if it fractures, whether caries is involved or not, as a fractured tooth may also become sensitive to hot and cold food or cause soft tissue trauma to areas within the oral cavity.

The filling procedure's purpose is to restore the tooth to its normal function ultimately, and this involves the elimination of any caries first, as well as the elimination of any discomfort or pain experienced by the patient.

The procedures discussed are:

- Amalgam fillings
- Composite fillings
- Glass ionomer fillings

BACKGROUND INFORMATION OF PROCEDURE – AMALGAM FILLINGS

Amalgam is a metallic material used for fillings, produced by mixing of an alloy powder (mainly silver) with a small amount of liquid mercury. This produces a malleable material that can be inserted fully into the tooth cavity and then carved into the shape of the tooth

Basic Guide to Dental Procedures, Third Edition. Carole Hollins.
© 2024 John Wiley & Sons Ltd. Published 2024 by John Wiley & Sons Ltd.

surface. Once set, it forms a solid plug in the cavity that is hard enough to chew on, as well as sealing the tooth's sensitive inner layers from further exposure to hot and cold stimulants present in foods and drinks.

As the material is metallic in appearance, it tends not to be used for anterior fillings as far more acceptable aesthetic substances are produced for use here, using tooth-coloured filling materials.

However, following the international decision to reduce the presence of toxic mercury in the environment worldwide in 2017, it is likely that dental amalgam will be gradually phased out as a filling material over the next few decades. Its use as a restorative in children under 15 years is already banned in the United Kingdom, but as it continues to be used for suitable cases in adult dental patients, details are included here for the sake of completeness.

DETAILS OF PROCEDURE – AMALGAM FILLINGS

The procedure is normally carried out under local anaesthetic so that the patient feels neither pain nor thermal stimulation in the tooth. The effects of the local anaesthetic wear off after several hours, by which time the dental treatment has been completed painlessly.

The instruments and materials required to administer a local anaesthetic are shown in Figure 3.9.

During the procedure, the dental nurse provides good moisture control in the oral cavity using high-speed suction equipment so the dentist has a clear field of vision at all times. The suction equipment removes saliva, debris from the tooth and water from the dental handpiece that cools the drill while in use.

The instruments and materials required to carry out an amalgam-filling procedure are shown in Figure 5.1.

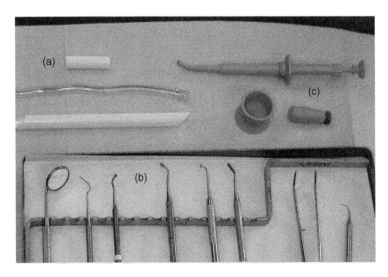

Figure 5.1 Instruments and materials for amalgam filling procedure. (a) Moisture control items. (b) Hand instruments. (c) Amalgam capsule, well and carrier

TOOTH RESTORATION WITH FILLINGS

TECHNIQUE:

- The dentist, nurse and patient wear personal protective equipment for safety reasons, and this usually consists of goggles and mask for the dental team and a protective bib and safety glasses for the patient (see Figure 3.6)
- Local anaesthetic is administered and allowed to take full effect
- As far as is safely possible without breaching the pulp chamber, the caries is removed from the tooth cavity using a combination of high and low-speed dental handpieces with drills and occasionally with the additional use of cutting hand instruments
- This produces a firm tooth cavity surface into which the filling can be placed, which is then undercut to prevent loss of the completed filling
- Depending on the depth of the finished cavity, a protective lining may be placed over its base so that the pulp beneath is not exposed to thermal irritation through the metallic filling
- In deeper cavities, more modern lining materials can be used, which act to stimulate the dentine layer to repair itself after caries removal so that a bridge of new tissue is formed over the pulp chamber, helping to prevent post-restorative sensitivity and pain
- The walls of the cavity can also be sealed using a light-cured resin-type material, which improves the tooth resistance to thermal stimulation and assists in reducing marginal leakage of the set filling
- If more than one tooth surface has been destroyed by caries, a metal matrix band is placed around the tooth and tightened to allow the amalgam to be pushed into the cavity from one surface without it squeezing out of the other
- The mixed amalgam is inserted into the cavity in increments by the dental team, starting at its deepest point and gradually filling the cavity to the surface of the tooth
- After each increment, the dentist uses hand instruments to push the plastic amalgam material into all the cavity depths so that no voids remain – these air spaces weaken the filling and allow future fracture, if present
- The dental nurse uses high-speed suction to remove all excess amalgam from the area as the dentist carves and shapes the surface of the filling
- Once completed, the shaping of the filling should allow the patient to bite together without prematurely contacting it, but so that the tooth can still be used for chewing
- The patient is advised not to attempt chewing until the local anaesthetic has worn off; otherwise, there is the risk of biting oneself
- By this time, the amalgam is hardened and fully set (Figure 5.2)

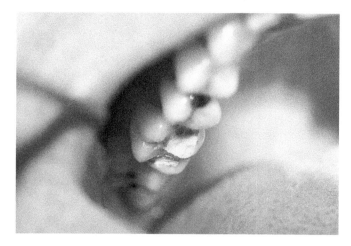

Figure 5.2 Completed amalgam filling in first molar tooth

BACKGROUND INFORMATION OF PROCEDURE – COMPOSITE FILLINGS

Composite is a tooth-coloured filling material available in many shades to match a wide range of tooth colours. It can be polished, once set, to produce a shiny surface that matches tooth enamel superbly and is, therefore, an excellent material to be used for anterior fillings. Many modern types of composite are also strong and wear-resistant enough to be used as a posterior filling material instead of amalgam. More recently, a new type of composite is available which changes colour to that of the surrounding tooth while setting, so that just one material can be used to restore any tooth shade rather than having to keep a range of materials of differing shades and matching each one (Figure 5.3).

Unlike amalgam, composite is not freshly mixed and then allowed to set with time, but rather it is used in its ready-mixed plastic state to fill a cavity, then set (or cured) by exposure to a blue curing lamp. This gives the dentist more time to fully adapt the plastic material to the tooth as required before using the curing lamp to harden it in a controlled manner.

Although composite is far superior to amalgam aesthetically, it can take longer, and the procedure is technique-sensitive. In addition, only certain types of composite are strong enough to be used in larger cavities in posterior teeth, as the chewing forces generated here are considerable.

DETAILS OF PROCEDURE – COMPOSITE FILLINGS

Again, local anaesthesia is usually administered before dental treatment begins, and a dental nurse provides moisture control throughout the procedure, as composite is particularly sensitive to moisture contamination from saliva, blood or irrigation water.

Indeed, some dentists choose to isolate the tooth completely from the rest of the oral cavity while placing composite fillings using a rubber dam. This allows the tooth to be

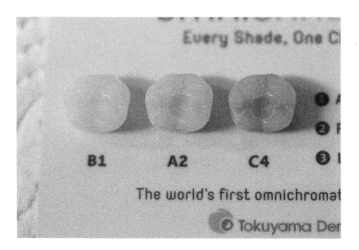

Figure 5.3 Omnichroma composite showing shade adaptation

TOOTH RESTORATION WITH FILLINGS

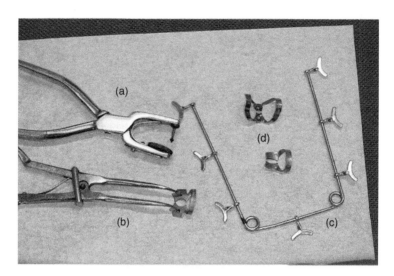

Figure 5.4 Rubber dam instruments. (a) Dam punch. (b) Dam clamp forceps, with clamp. (c) Dam frame. (d) Selection of other clamps

restored to project through the rubber dam sheet while keeping all other oral structures away, thus preventing saliva contamination of the tooth while the filling is placed.

The instruments required to apply a rubber dam to a tooth are shown in Figure 5.4.

The equipment and materials required to carry out a composite filling procedure are shown in Figure 5.5.

TECHNIQUE:

- The dentist, nurse and patient wear personal protective equipment, and ideally, the patient's safety glasses are orange-tinted to counteract the blue curing lamp
- Local anaesthetic is administered and allowed to take full effect
- A rubber dam is placed if required (Figure 5.6)
- As much caries as possible is removed from the tooth cavity without breaching the pulp chamber as before, but then the preparation can be minimal as the composite material bonds to enamel and no undercuts are required to hold the filling in place
- A lining may be placed in deeper cavities to prevent chemical irritation of the pulp by the filling material
- The required shade is chosen using a shade guide in natural light (this may be taken beforehand if a rubber dam is placed)
- Alternatively, a universal composite material can be used that adapts to the colour of the tooth during curing
- The exposed enamel edges of the cavity are covered in acid etch to chemically roughen their surfaces
- The etch is washed off, the edges dried, and then unfilled resin is wiped over them and cured with the blue lamp for a short time to produce a sticky layer of material

- The resin forms a bond between the enamel and the filling material, locking the latter into place
- A transparent matrix strip is used to avoid overspill as the composite is placed into the cavity in 2 mm increments that are individually cured to ensure full setting of the overall filling
- Alternatively, a 'bulk flow' composite can be used to fill the majority of the cavity in one cure, then the uppermost layer of ordinary composite is shade-matched and used as a 'topping' to complete the restoration – this is a faster technique overall and is useful with larger restorations
- The matrix is transparent to allow the curing light beam to pass through it
- Coloured articulating paper is used to identify any premature contacts on any biting surfaces of the filling, and these are removed to allow the patients to achieve their correct bite
- Polishing strips, discs and burs are used to produce the final shiny surface of the completed filling (Figure 5.7 shows an old composite filling, as a new one is very difficult to see because of its superb aesthetics)
- Although the filling is fully set once cured, the patient is advised not to attempt chewing until the local anaesthetic has worn off to avoid soft tissue injury

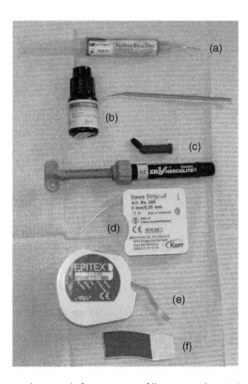

Figure 5.5 Equipment and materials for composite filling procedure. (a) Acid etchant. (b) Resin and applicator. (c) Composite material example. (d) Transparent matrix strip. (e) Finishing strip. (f) Articulating paper

TOOTH RESTORATION WITH FILLINGS

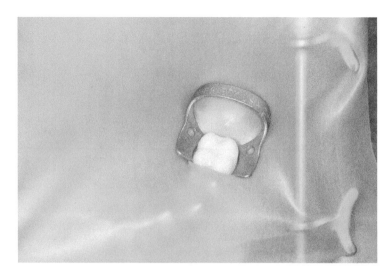

Figure 5.6 Rubber dam in place on lower molar tooth

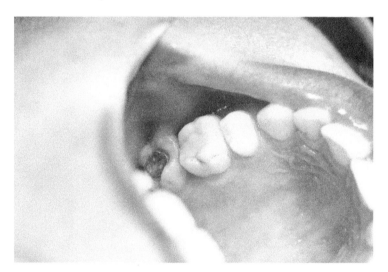

Figure 5.7 Completed composite filling – old filling shown in the first molar tooth as new filling is not easily visible

BACKGROUND INFORMATION OF PROCEDURE – GLASS IONOMER FILLINGS

Glass ionomer is another tooth-coloured filling material available for tooth restoration, although the shade range is more limited than composite. It is also less translucent and cannot be polished to give a shiny surface, so the final aesthetics produced are inferior to those achieved with composite materials.

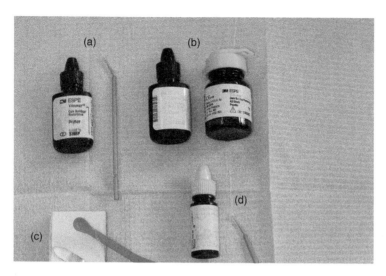

Figure 5.8 Equipment and materials for glass ionomer filling procedure. (a) Conditioning liquid and applicator. (b) Powder and liquid filling material example. (c) Waxed pad, spatula, and measuring scoop. (d) Varnish and applicator

The advantage of glass ionomer over other filling materials is that it is adhesive to all tooth surfaces – enamel, dentine and cementum – and is therefore invaluable in filling cavities where only minimal, if any, tooth preparation is possible. This is a particular advantage when filling abrasion cavities produced at the necks of the teeth, often by overzealous toothbrushing by the patient.

Glass ionomer materials are also useful in filling the deciduous teeth of young patients who often do not tolerate the administration of local anaesthetic. They are of special value here as they release fluoride into the cavity and help to slow or stop the progression of the caries.

The material is usually provided as a powder of glass-like material to be mixed by hand with an acidic liquid or as a capsule containing both to be mixed mechanically; some set chemically with time, while others set after exposure to the blue curing lamp. Attempts to adjust the surface of the filling once set produce a chalky appearance, so accurate placement of a light-cure type requiring no adjustment produces the best aesthetic result.

The equipment and materials required to carry out a glass ionomer filling procedure are shown in Figure 5.8.

DETAILS OF PROCEDURE – GLASS IONOMER FILLINGS

As little or no tooth preparation is required with this material unless caries is present, local anaesthesia may not always be required. However, good moisture control is imperative to the filling setting properly, so a rubber dam may well be placed in adult patients.

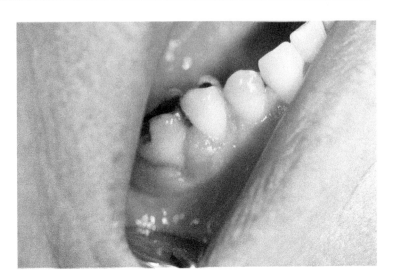

Figure 5.9 Completed glass ionomer filling on the exposed root of lower molar

TECHNIQUE:

- The dentist, nurse and patient wear personal protective equipment
- Local anaesthetic is administered if caries removal is necessary
- A rubber dam is placed if required
- Caries is removed as far as possible if present; otherwise, no tooth preparation is required
- The cavity is conditioned by wiping it over fully with polyacrylic liquid to remove dirt and any preparation debris and allow chemical bonding of the filling to the tooth
- The conditioner is washed off, and the cavity is dried
- Deeper cavities are lined to prevent chemical irritation of the pulp
- The mixed filling material is applied and fully adapted to the cavity so that no adjustment is required once set
- Light-cured types of glass ionomer are cured as necessary, while chemically cured types are kept dry while setting occurs with time
- The set surface is coated with a waterproof varnish to prevent the filling from drying out once set (Figure 5.9)

AFTERCARE OF FILLINGS

No matter how well placed, microscopically, the edges of a filling provide a new surface area for plaque and oral bacteria to adhere to, giving the potential for further carious attack if not removed regularly.

Consistently high standards of oral hygiene must be maintained by the patient to prevent this from happening, especially interdentally if the filling extends between the teeth. This involves using a good toothbrushing technique with a good quality fluoridated toothpaste, as well as using interdental brushes to clean regularly and effectively between the teeth (see Figure 2.16). Dental tape or floss can also be used to dislodge food debris from between the teeth if necessary (see Figure 2.13). Ideally, a plaque-suppressing mouthwash should also be used routinely to help control the amount of plaque build-up that occurs.

The standard of oral hygiene achieved should be monitored and reinforced as necessary at regular dental examinations. Where techniques are poor, and calculus has developed, this should be fully removed by scaling and polishing the teeth.

Patients should also be advised to alter their diet when they have experienced caries previously. Their intake of foods and drinks high in free sugars or acids should be reduced as far as possible and confined to mealtimes to allow the natural buffering action of saliva to minimise any carious attack.

Failure to comply with these oral health instructions will likely result in further caries and the need for further fillings in the future.

Chapter 6

Tooth restoration with crowns, bridges, veneers or inlays

REASON FOR PROCEDURE – CROWNS

Each time a tooth is restored with a filling, some of the tooth tissue is removed. Eventually, this compromises the strength of the remaining tooth, and it may begin to fracture under normal occlusal forces. This especially occurs when teeth have been root treated, so it is usual for heavily filled and root-filled teeth to be crowned before fracture occurs.

In other cases, a tooth may be poorly shaped and require elective crowning to be more aesthetically pleasing. Similarly, a tooth may be too poorly shaped to assist in the retention of, say, a denture, but can be made so by elective crowning.

BACKGROUND INFORMATION OF PROCEDURE – CROWNS

Posterior crowns are sometimes constructed from non-precious or precious metals such as yellow gold. These metallic materials provide maximum strength to withstand occlusal forces and have no fracture risk. More modern posterior crowns and anterior crowns are made of either tooth-coloured ceramic throughout, or have porcelain bonded to a substructure of metal, and these both give an aesthetically pleasing result when shaded and matched accurately with the adjacent teeth. Although modern techniques of crown construction are superb, it is possible for ceramic crowns to fracture or to break away from their metallic substructure so that repairs or even replacements are required. This can occur in patients with especially heavy bites or in those who grind their teeth.

DETAILS OF PROCEDURE – CROWNS

Unless the tooth to be crowned has been root treated and is therefore non-vital, crown preparation is usually carried out under local anaesthetic so that the patient feels neither pain nor thermal stimulation in the tooth throughout the procedure. The equipment and materials required to administer local anaesthetic are shown in Figure 3.9.

Basic Guide to Dental Procedures, Third Edition. Carole Hollins.
© 2024 John Wiley & Sons Ltd. Published 2024 by John Wiley & Sons Ltd.

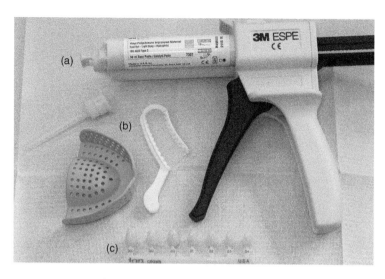

Figure 6.1 Equipment and materials for crown preparation procedure. (a) Elastomer-based impression material example. (b) Selection of impression trays. (c) Temporary crown form example

During the preparation procedure, a dental nurse provides good moisture control in the oral cavity using high-speed suction equipment. This provides a clear field of vision for the dentist, as well as makes the patient more comfortable by removing water, saliva and tooth debris from the mouth while the tooth is prepared.

The prepared tooth requires thermal protection after the procedure by being covered with a temporary crown material such as acrylic, as the permanent crown has to be individually constructed by a technician before it can be fitted, a process that usually takes several days. Alternatively, an intraoral scanner can be used to send details of the prepared tooth to a milling machine on the premises, and the crown can be constructed by the machine and ready for cementation within the hour. The instruments required to carry out a crown preparation procedure are the same as those used for filling and are shown in Figure 5.1b.

The equipment and materials required to carry out a crown preparation procedure are shown in Figure 6.1.

TECHNIQUE:

- The dentist, nurse and patient wear personal protective equipment, as usual
- Local anaesthetic is administered and allowed to take full effect
- The shade and shape of the crown are chosen by the dentist and patient using a shade guide (Figure 6.2)
- A rubber dam is placed if required
- All sides and the occlusal surface of the tooth are reduced by a uniform amount using a bur in the high-speed handpiece, so that space is created for the crown to be constructed and fitted over the remaining tooth without altering the patient's occlusion
- The side reduction is completed to produce a near parallel tooth core, to give maximum retention of the crown on cementation (Figure 6.3)

(continued)

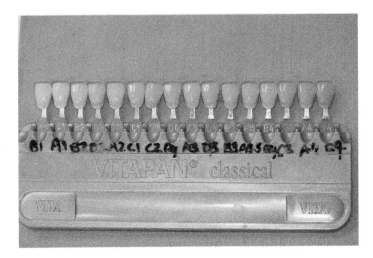

Figure 6.2 Example of crown shade guide

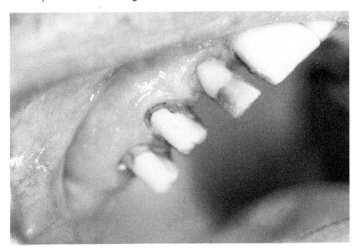

Figure 6.3 Three upper right teeth prepared for a crown procedure

TECHNIQUE: (*Continued*)

- Once the tooth preparation is complete, impressions are taken of both arches and the patient's normal biting position is also recorded – this allows the technician to put the models together during crown construction and ensure that the occlusion has not been altered by the crown
- Impression of the opposing arch can be taken in alginate, but that of the working arch has to be in a very accurate, non-tearing elastomeric material such as silicone or polyether
- When satisfactory impressions have been produced, the tooth core is coated with a temporary acrylic material or fitted with a temporary crown form to prevent sensitivity and to restore some degree of aesthetics while the permanent crown is constructed (Figure 6.4)
- Once the crown has been constructed, the patient reattends for its cementation

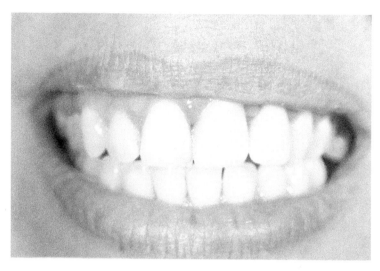

Figure 6.4 Temporary crowns in place on the upper left incisors

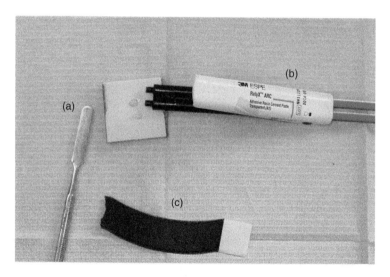

Figure 6.5 Equipment and materials for crown cementation procedure. (a) Mixing pad and spatula. (b) Dual-cure luting material example. (c) Articulating paper

The equipment and materials required to cement a permanent crown are shown in Figure 6.5.

- Again, local anaesthetic is administered, and a rubber dam is placed if required
- On removal of the temporary material, the crown is tried onto the tooth core and checked for accuracy of fit, shade and occlusion
- If satisfactory, the crown is cemented permanently onto the tooth core using one of a variety of luting cements (Figure 6.6)

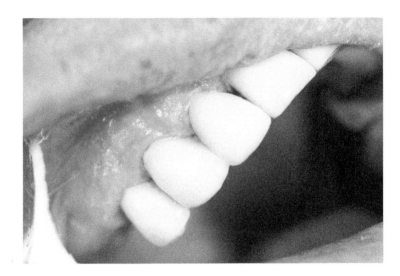

Figure 6.6 Cemented crowns on three upper right teeth

AFTERCARE OF CROWNS

As with fillings, microscopically, all fixed prosthetic restorations provide a surface area for the attachment of plaque and oral bacteria. As crown margins are deliberately placed at the gingival margin to give superior aesthetics, any plaque accumulation on the margins can potentially cause either caries of the underlying tooth core or periodontal disease down the root of the tooth.

A consistently high standard of oral hygiene around crown margins is therefore imperative. This involves good toothbrushing using good quality fluoride toothpaste and successful interdental cleaning using interdental brushes, floss or tape. However, as some crowns are placed specifically to reduce the space between adjacent teeth and prevent food trapping, it is possible that only the finest of interdental brush sizes can be used effectively. The dental team will assist and advise the patient with regard to interdental cleaning.

Regular use of a plaque-suppressing mouthwash should also be encouraged, and the oral hygiene standard achieved by the patient can be monitored and reinforced at regular dental examinations. Any calculus found to be present should be fully removed by scaling and polishing the teeth.

As always, a diet high in sugars and acids should be reduced to an absolute minimum and confined to mealtimes.

BACKGROUND INFORMATION OF PROCEDURE – BRIDGES

A bridge is a multi-unit fixed restoration used to replace one or a few missing teeth in a dental arch. However, in advanced cases, multiple bridges can be fitted to provide full-mouth rehabilitation.

Various designs of bridges are available, and which are used in each case has to be determined by the dentist on its merits.

For patients with only a few missing teeth and a low biting force in the area of the bridge, a minimal amount of tooth preparation can be carried out, and an acid etch retained bridge can be placed. Where occlusal forces are likely to dislodge this type of restoration, a more conventional design is used, where the adjacent teeth are prepared crowns, and the missing teeth are incorporated into the whole multi-unit structure.

Bridges are usually constructed of porcelain bonded to a metallic substructure, although some modern, all ceramic materials are also available, as for single unit crowns.

DETAILS OF PROCEDURE – BRIDGES

As minimal tooth preparation is carried out for an acid etch bridge preparation, it is often unnecessary for a local anaesthetic to be administered. With more conventional designs involving whole tooth preparation, it is usual for a local anaesthetic to be administered for any vital teeth involved.

As always, a dental nurse provides good moisture control in the oral cavity throughout the bridge preparation procedure.

The instruments, equipment and materials required for a bridge preparation are as those detailed previously for a crown preparation (see Figures 5.1b and 6.1).

TECHNIQUE:

- The dentist, nurse and patient wear personal protective equipment
- Local anaesthetic is administered if necessary and allowed to take full effect
- The design of the bridge will have been discussed and determined previously, and the shade is now chosen
- A rubber dam is placed if required
- If an acid etch bridge is being provided, a small area of enamel at the back of the retaining adjacent teeth is removed to provide room for the technician to construct the retaining metal wings to hold the bridge in place
- These have to be constructed so as not to interfere with the patient's normal occlusion
- When a more conventional bridge is being provided, each retaining tooth is reduced to a core as for crown preparation, using the same technique and design principles (see Figure 6.3)
- Once prepared, an impression of the working arch is taken in a highly accurate material such as silicone or polyether, and one of the opposing arch is taken in alginate
- The bite and jaw movements can be recorded simply, or with the help of articulated study models, depending on the complexity of the case
- The prepared teeth are temporarily covered to prevent sensitivity after the preparation procedure is completed, as with crown preparations
- In complex cases, the metallic substructure of the bridge (if used) is tried for accuracy of fit before the porcelain is bonded to it, as this avoids costly full remakes if problems do occur
- Once the bridge is fully constructed, the patient reattends for its cementation

The equipment and materials required to cement a bridge are for crown cementation and are shown in Figure 6.5.

- Local anaesthetic is administered, and a rubber dam is placed as necessary
- On removal of the temporary coverings, the bridge is tried onto the retaining teeth and checked for accuracy of fit, shade and occlusion
- The replaced missing tooth (or teeth) is checked for its fit against the bony ridge of the dental arch to ensure that the area can be easily cleaned by the patient
- Once satisfactory, an acid etch retained bridge is cemented using one of a variety of light-cured bonding materials
- A conventional bridge is cemented using one of a variety of luting cements

AFTERCARE OF BRIDGES

All of the aftercare advice for crowns similarly applies to bridges, but additional oral hygiene techniques also need to be employed when maintaining the pontic areas of a bridge. The pontic is the section of the bridge that replaces the missing tooth or teeth, and rests on the ridge of the dental arch once the bridge is cemented.

The point where the pontic rests on the gingiva is a difficult area to clean and may accumulate plaque and oral bacteria quite easily. This causes gingival inflammation unless the plaque is removed, either by vigorous mouth washing or by physically cleaning the underside of the pontic using floss or tape.

Where the pontic has retainers on both sides so that the bridge is a solid structure, superfloss can be threaded beneath the pontic and used to clean its underside. Superfloss has a stiff end for threading as described, which is attached to an expanded spongy section that then runs into normal floss (Figure 6.7). It has been designed specifically to clean bridges in this way.

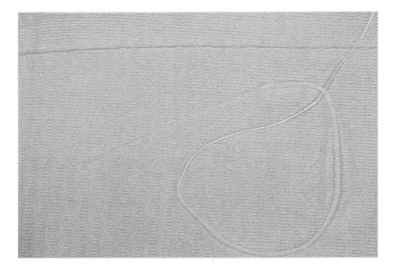

Figure 6.7 Superfloss for cleaning beneath a bridge pontic

BACKGROUND INFORMATION OF PROCEDURE – VENEERS

A less invasive technique than conventional crown preparation for improving the aesthetics of a tooth is to place veneers. These are thin layers of porcelain or composite/acrylic-type material that are acid etch cemented to the front surface of any number of anterior teeth, to improve a patient's appearance by correcting dark or mal-aligned teeth, or both.

They have no other functional purpose than a cosmetic one, and their fragility and ease of fracture or loss dictate their case suitability. Patients with aberrant occlusal habits (such as nail biting, pen biting, or using the teeth as tools) or those with heavy bites (clenchers/grinders) are usually unsuitable for veneers, particularly those made of porcelain, which tend to be more fragile than composite/acrylic materials.

A patient with well-aligned but discoloured anterior teeth may also undergo professional tooth whitening to improve their appearance, rather than undergo the relatively invasive procedure of having porcelain veneers fitted (see Chapter 13).

DETAILS OF PROCEDURE – VENEERS

As minimal tooth preparation is carried out for a veneer, it is often unnecessary for a local anaesthetic to be administered. Indeed, it is frequently root-filled, discoloured teeth that have veneers placed to improve aesthetics, as full crown preparations on these teeth can sometimes compromise them enough to cause fracture with time.

A dental nurse provides good moisture control in the oral cavity throughout the veneer preparation procedure.

The instruments, equipment, and materials required for a veneer preparation are similar to those required for a crown preparation procedure, as shown in Figures 5.1b and 6.1, although a temporary crown form is unnecessary in veneer cases.

TOOTH RESTORATION WITH CROWNS, BRIDGES, VENEERS OR INLAYS

TECHNIQUE:

- The dentist, nurse and patient wear personal protective equipment
- Local anaesthetic is administered as necessary, and allowed to take full effect
- The shade and shape of the veneer are chosen by the dentist and patient, and the need for any opaquing technique, if a particularly dark tooth is involved, is decided upon
- This may be necessary to prevent the tooth discolouration from being visible through the thin porcelain or composite/acrylic veneer once fitted
- A rubber dam is placed if required (see Figure 5.4)
- The labial (front) surface of each tooth to be veneered is reduced uniformly using a bur in the high-speed handpiece (Figure 6.8)
- This is to provide the technician with sufficient space to construct the veneer so that the restoration remains in line with the adjacent teeth rather than projecting further forwards than required
- Once the veneer preparation is complete, a highly accurate working impression is taken in a material such as silicone or polyether
- If the occlusion of the prepared tooth has been altered, then an opposing alginate impression and bite record are also taken

(continued)

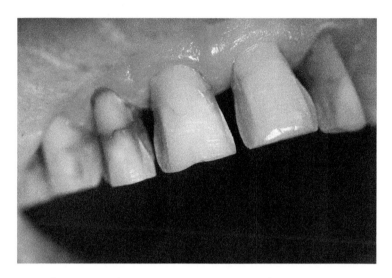

Figure 6.8 Tooth preparation for veneers on upper anterior teeth

TECHNIQUE: (*Continued*)

- The prepared tooth surface can be temporarily covered with glass ionomer or restorative composite to avoid sensitivity and improve aesthetics, but this is sometimes not carried out with non-vital teeth
- Once the veneer has been constructed, the patient reattends for its cementation

The equipment and materials required to cement a veneer are shown in Figure 6.9.

- Local anaesthetic is administered, and a rubber dam is placed if required
- On removal of any temporary covering placed, the veneer is placed onto the tooth and checked for accuracy of fit, shade and shape
- The final shade can be accurately achieved by the use of various tooth-coloured luting cements, if necessary
- The veneer is secured to the tooth using one of a variety of light-cured bonding materials (Figures 6.10 and 6.11)

AFTERCARE OF VENEERS

As with other restorations, veneers can be subject to plaque and oral bacteria accumulations at their margins. Their aftercare advice is similar to crowns, whereby a consistently good standard of plaque removal is required to prevent caries developing at the veneer margins and periodontal problems developing at the gingival margins.

This is achieved using a thorough toothbrushing technique with fluoride toothpaste, careful interdental cleaning using floss, tape or interdental brush where space allows, and the regular use of a plaque-suppressing mouthwash.

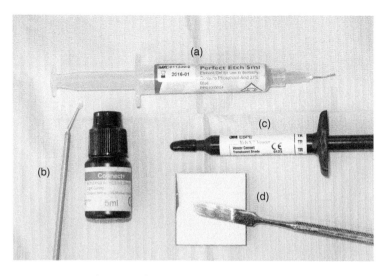

Figure 6.9 Equipment and materials for veneer cementation procedure. (a) Acid etchant. (b) Resin and applicator. (c) Veneer luting cement example. (d) Mixing pad and spatula

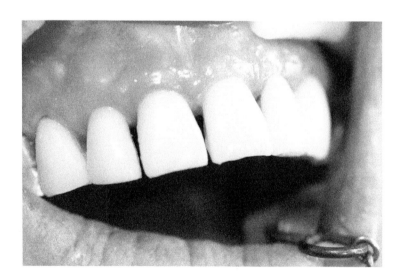

Figure 6.10 Cemented porcelain veneers on upper anterior teeth

Regular dental examinations should be carried out, where oral hygiene techniques can be reinforced as necessary, as well as any scaling and polishing carried out to remove any accumulated calculus deposits.

Diet advice includes reducing intake of sugars and acids to a minimum, as well as for them to be confined to mealtimes only.

Patients should also be warned of the potential fragility of veneers in certain circumstances. Actions such as biting fingernails and habits such as holding pens in the mouth

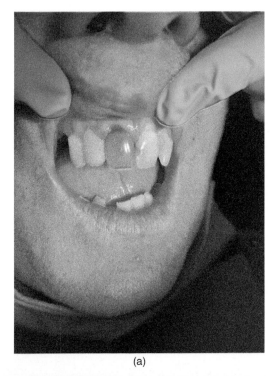

(a)

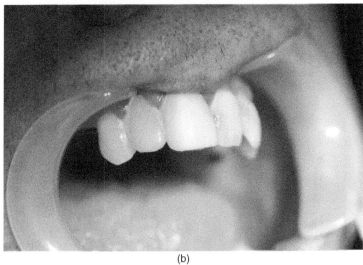

(b)

Figure 6.11 Composite veneer treatment of upper right discoloured tooth (a) Before. (b) After.

may be sufficient to crack a porcelain veneer and require its removal and remake. Patients should always be discouraged from these habits and activities anyway, as they are often sufficient to splinter fillings and slivers of enamel from the teeth.

REASON FOR PROCEDURE – INLAYS

An inlay is a device used to fill a prepared cavity in a tooth with a solid, pre-formed material rather than with a more conventional malleable filling material that can be manipulated into shape before setting, such as composite, glass ionomer or amalgam. The advantage of using an inlay in this situation is the greater strength of the material used versus that of conventional fill-ing materials. This is particularly important in patients with a very strong bite or in patients who habitually grind their teeth, as they tend to suffer from an increased incidence of filling fractures.

The inclusion of inlays in this chapter rather than with fillings is due to the similarity in the method of tooth preparation required as well as the materials available for inlay construction, both features being similar to those for crown and bridge work.

BACKGROUND INFORMATION OF PROCEDURE – INLAYS

As with crowns and bridges, inlays are conventionally constructed indirectly in a labora-tory rather than at the chair side, using materials such as precious and non-precious metal alloys and ceramics. More modern systems are now available where intraoral scanners and in-house milling machines can be used to construct the inlay on the premises and within the hour.

Inlays are usually placed in posterior teeth, which undergo heavy occlusal forces dur-ing normal chewing actions. These forces may be strong enough to fracture large conven-tional fillings and allow caries to recur in the affected tooth through the fracture. Small, uncomplicated cavities do not usually warrant the extra time and expense of restoring them with an inlay, and their use in anterior teeth has also declined with the development of more aesthetic anterior filling materials.

DETAILS OF PROCEDURE – INLAYS

Unless the tooth receiving the inlay has been root treated and is therefore non-vital, inlay preparation is usually carried out under local anaesthetic so that the patient feels neither pain nor thermal stimulation in the tooth throughout the procedure.

While the inlay is being constructed in the laboratory by the technician, a temporary filling material is placed to seal the cavity and prevent any food packing from occurring in it, as well as to protect the tooth from any uncomfortable thermal stimulation.

During the preparation procedure, a dental nurse provides good moisture control in the oral cavity using high-speed suction equipment. This provides a clear field of vision for the dentist, as well as makes the patient more comfortable by removing water, saliva and tooth debris from the mouth during the preparation procedure.

The instruments required to carry out an inlay preparation procedure are the same as those used for a filling procedure, as shown in Figure 5.1b.

The same impression and bite recording techniques are used for crown or bridge preparation procedures. The only additional equipment and material required is for mixing and placing a temporary filling material to seal the cavity while the inlay is constructed.

TECHNIQUE:

- The dentist, nurse and patient wear personal protective equipment
- Local anaesthetic is administered as necessary, and allowed to take full effect
- The material used to construct the inlay is decided previously by the dentist and the patient, and if a ceramic material is to be used, the shade is chosen
- A rubber dam is placed if required (see Figure 5.4)
- Any existing filling is removed using ordinary cavity preparation burs in the high-speed handpiece
- Similarly, any carious tooth tissue is removed down to sound dentine to leave a hollowed-out cavity within the tooth of varying shape and size dependent on the amount of caries removed
- The inner walls of the cavity must now be prepared to produce a near-parallel shape, by the infilling of any undercuts with an adhesive restorative material such as composite or glass ionomer
- The walls must be near-parallel to allow the inlay to be seated accurately, while providing maximum retention to prevent its inadvertent dislodgement during function
- In some cases, the preparation is extended over one or more cusps of the tooth for improved tooth protection and functionality and is then referred to as an inlay/onlay preparation (see Figure 6.12)
- Once the inlay preparation is complete, a highly accurate working impression is taken in a material such as silicone or polyether
- An opposing alginate impression and bite record are also taken so that the technician can construct the inlay surface to fit neatly into the occlusion
- The inlay cavity is then temporarily filled while the inlay is being constructed by the technician
- Once the inlay has been constructed, the patient reattends for its cementation
- Alternatively, the completed inlay preparation is intraorally scanned at the chair side and the inlay milled in-house within the hour, while the patient remains in the dental chair with the tooth remaining under local anaesthetic

The equipment and materials required to cement an inlay are the same as for a crown cementation, as shown in Figure 6.5.

- Local anaesthetic is administered, and a rubber dam is placed if required
- The temporary filling material is carefully drilled out of the cavity without altering the shape at all
- The inlay is placed in the cavity to ensure it seats fully, fills the cavity to the margins fully and sits accurately in the occlusion (Figure 6.12)
- Once satisfactory, the inlay is cemented into the cavity using a conventional luting cement or a dual-cure cement
- A final check is made of the seated restoration, using articulating paper to highlight any premature contacts

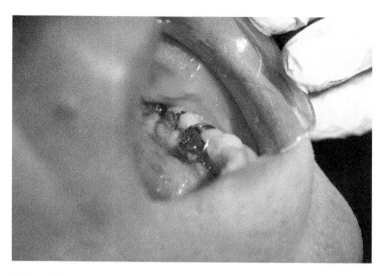

Figure 6.12 Gold inlay/onlay cemented in lower left molar tooth

AFTERCARE OF INLAYS

As with other restorations, inlays can be subject to plaque and oral bacteria accumulations at their margins. Many inlays also involve extensions into the interdental areas of the dental arch to replace contact points between teeth, which are particularly difficult regions to clean in the oral cavity. Consequently, in addition to the usual oral hygiene advice of effective and regular brushing using fluoride toothpaste, these patients should also be advised to carry out regular interdental cleaning, using floss or tape or a recommended size and design of interdental brush (see Figure 2.14).

The restoration is routinely checked for any signs of marginal leakage at each recall appointment, visually and manually. Where the inlay extends into the interdental areas, radiographs can be taken as required to check these areas for leakage and caries formation in the same way as conventional fillings are checked and monitored.

Diet advice includes reducing intake of sugars and acids to a minimum, as well as for these products to be confined to mealtimes only.

Chapter 7

Tooth restoration with endodontic techniques

REASON FOR PROCEDURE

Any event that results in the pulp tissue within the root canal of a tooth being at risk of inflammation or infection may eventually lead to the death of that tooth. Once a tooth has died, it is a source of either painless chronic infection or acute and very painful infection – neither of which is amenable to the oral health of a patient.

Events that can occur resulting in the inflammation of the pulp (pulpitis) include the following:

- Deep caries lying close to, or exposing, the pulp
- Thermal injury, from the use of hand pieces without cooling irrigation, for example
- Chemical irritation from some restorative materials in deep restorations
- Trauma, which may have been severe enough to cause tooth fracture in some cases
- Prolonged irritation of the pulp tissue from very deep fillings within the tooth, which may easily transmit thermal and pressure shocks

The method available to the dentist for removing the symptoms and treating the tooth to save it from extraction is one of the following endodontic techniques:

- Pulp capping, either indirect or direct
- Pulpotomy in both immature and mature permanent teeth
- Pulpectomy (conventional root canal treatment)

Occasionally, a successful root-filled tooth may develop problems at a later date (sometimes years later) and result in a recurrent infection at the end of the root. This may be treated and the tooth saved from extraction by either a re-root filling procedure or a surgical procedure called an apicectomy.

Basic Guide to Dental Procedures, Third Edition. Carole Hollins.
© 2024 John Wiley & Sons Ltd. Published 2024 by John Wiley & Sons Ltd.

BACKGROUND INFORMATION OF PROCEDURE – PULP CAPPING

Conventionally, this was a technique carried out as a temporary measure to stabilise the tooth before proceeding to either pulpotomy or pulpectomy to save it from extraction. More recently, and with the advent of modern calcium silicate cements for use in the field of endodontics, pulp capping is now usually carried out as a permanent procedure under the following circumstances:

- Indirect pulp capping – mild and short-lived symptoms of pulpitis with no carious pulpal exposure present
- Direct pulp capping – mild and short-lived symptoms of pulpitis with minimal carious or traumatic pulpal exposure present in an apparently vital pulp

Indirect pulp capping aims to remove as much caries without exposing the pulp, then place one of the modern bioactive calcium silicate cements (Figure 7.1) in the base of the cavity to allow the pulpitis symptoms to subside as the inflammation resolves. With direct pulp capping, the cement contents also allow the tooth to form a bridge of new tissue over the exposure site, so that the vital pulp is protected and retained as the inflammation resolves. The procedure for indirect pulp capping is a typical restorative procedure, as detailed in Chapter 5, with the additional stage of placing the bioactive calcium silicate material in the deepest part of the cavity before placing the final restoration above it.

DETAILS OF PROCEDURE – DIRECT PULP CAPPING

If the pulp exposure occurred during restorative treatment, it is likely that a local anaesthetic has already been administered. If a recent trauma has caused the exposure, the tooth is likely to be concussed and unresponsive to stimulation; therefore, not requiring a local anaesthetic procedure to be carried out in some cases.

In any event, the tooth must be kept as clean as possible and isolated from the oral cavity to prevent the introduction of microorganisms into the pulp chamber.

TECHNIQUE:

- The dentist, nurse and patient wear personal protective equipment
- Local anaesthetic is administered if required
- The tooth is isolated from any saliva contamination using appropriate moisture control techniques
- At the exposure site, a vital pulp will appear as a small pink/red spot with little, if any, bleeding present
- Any bleeding is arrested using sterile cotton wool pledgets, possibly soaked in a local anaesthetic solution containing a vasoconstrictor such as adrenaline
- Once bleeding has been arrested (this should be achieved in less than 5 minutes) and the area is dry, a layer of the pre-mixed calcium silicate cement is placed to completely cover the exposure site and the floor of the cavity
- Once the cement is set, the remaining cavity or fracture site is then restored with a conventional filling material, as discussed in Chapter 5.

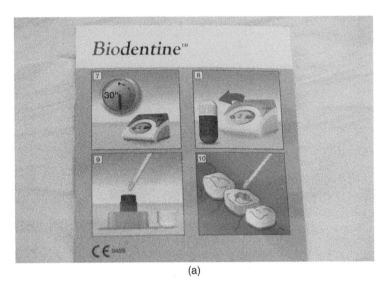

(a)

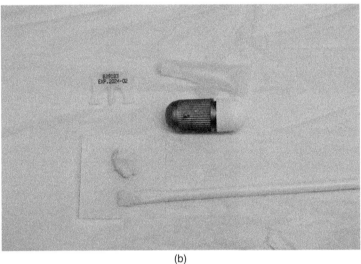

(b)

Figure 7.1 Example of a bioactive calcium silicate cement material. (a) Mixing instructions for product. (b) Mixed material ready for use

BACKGROUND INFORMATION OF PROCEDURE – PULPOTOMY OF IMMATURE TEETH

The partial removal of pulp tissue from the pulp chamber in the crown of the tooth only, and not that extending into the root canal, is called pulpotomy.

When trauma occurs to a permanent tooth in a young patient, it is often the case that the root canal is still wide open at the apex as the root is still growing – this can be determined by taking a radiograph. On average, a root continues to grow, and the apex closes for up to 3 years after the tooth has erupted.

When an open apex is present, the tooth often does not die as a result of the trauma, as the wide apex ensures that a good blood supply to the pulp is maintained during the inflammatory process and pulpal death is avoided. In these cases, only the potentially infected part of the pulp at the exposure site needs to be removed, while the apical blood supply ensures that the remainder of the pulp tissue heals itself and allows root formation and apex closure to continue.

BACKGROUND INFORMATION OF PROCEDURE – PULPOTOMY OF MATURE TEETH

- Evidence has emerged over the last decade that many mature permanent teeth suffering from carious exposure with inflammation affecting just the pulp tissue in the tooth crown, and not the root(s), may also be successfully treated with a pulpotomy technique rather than full root canal treatment (pulpectomy)... The advantages of this procedure over a conventional pulpectomy procedure are as follows:
- Tooth remains vital and responsive to proprioception (touch, movement, sensations, etc.)
- Regenerative and repair potential of the remaining pulp tissue is retained and helps to prevent infection from occurring at the apex
- Structural integrity of the tooth is maintained, lowering the risk of tooth fracture in the future

DETAILS OF PROCEDURE – PULPOTOMY

As the pulp tissue is still vital, local anaesthetic is required for the procedure. It is important to the success of the technique that any risk of contamination of the remaining pulp tissue is kept to an absolute minimum, so the dental nurse provides good moisture control throughout.

Similar additional equipment and materials as those used for a pulp capping procedure are required.

TECHNIQUE:

- The dentist, nurse and patient wear personal protective equipment
- Local anaesthetic is administered and allowed to take full effect
- The tooth is isolated from saliva contamination, ideally using a rubber dam but this may not always be possible, especially for a young patient
- The tooth crown is cleaned and disinfected by wiping with an antiseptic such as chlorhexidine
- The pulp chamber is opened through the fracture site or exposure site using a sterile bur in the high-speed hand piece

(continued)

TECHNIQUE: (*Continued*)

- In the case of a carious exposure in a mature permanent tooth, all of the caries must be removed peripherally before accessing the exposure site to reduce the likelihood of further bacterial contamination
- The dentist assesses the health of the vital pulp visually to determine the likely success of the procedure; healthy pulp is uniformly pink, so darkened or discoloured pulp tissue will indicate infection is present and the procedure is more likely to fail
- The healthy pulp tissue, within the pulp chamber of the crown only, is separated from that in the root canal using a new sterile bur in the high-speed hand piece
- Any bleeding of the amputated pulp stump is arrested using sterile cotton wool pledgets soaked in medical bleach solution – bleeding should be arrested within 10 minutes if the pulpotomy is to be successful
- The presence of unhealthy pulp tissue, dead tissue, pus, or a failure to achieve haemostasis within 10 minutes are all indicators that a full root canal treatment procedure should be carried out, rather than a pulpotomy
- Otherwise, if bleeding is arrested within 10-minutes the dry pulp stump is covered and sealed over with a deep layer of a bioactive calcium silicate cement that assists the remaining pulp tissue to heal and resolves any inflammation
- The material also allows a protective bridge of tissue to form over the remaining pulp tissue with time, so that the tooth maintains its vitality
- The fracture site or cavity in the tooth is then restored to full function and aesthetics at the same appointment, using one of the permanent restorative filling materials available
- Following a waiting period of 3–6 months to determine if the pulpotomy procedure has been successful, a full coverage restoration such as a crown is advised to prolong the long-term survival of the tooth

BACKGROUND INFORMATION OF PROCEDURE – PULPECTOMY

When a mature permanent tooth undergoes an event causing pulpal inflammation with infection and necrosis extending into the pulp tissue of the root, the end result is usually the death of the tooth. The closed root apex of an adult tooth prevents adequate blood flow from helping to fight the inflammation and remove the excess fluids that build up during the inflammatory process. The ensuing swelling compresses the pulpal tissues within the root canal and tooth death occurs. An infection develops at the root apex that is referred to as a periapical abscess, which will be visible on a diagnostic X-ray as a circular radiolucency at the tip of the affected tooth root (Figure 7.2). If the infection develops quickly, it tends to be associated with facial swelling, an intraoral pus-filled swelling, and pain and is an acute abscess (Figure 7.3a and b), whereas a slowly developing chronic infection is often painless with no swelling, but often exhibits a discharging sinus tract, which is referred to as a 'gum boil' by patients (Figure 7.4).

The patient therefore experiences varying degrees of pain and swelling throughout the tooth death process, and only a successful pulpectomy procedure helps to avoid the extraction of the affected tooth.

The aim of pulpectomy, or root canal treatment, is to remove all the pulpal tissue from the tooth (both from the crown of the tooth and all the roots) and replace it with a sterile root-filling material. This material must fully seal the root canal and prevent any contamination from causing further infection at the root apex.

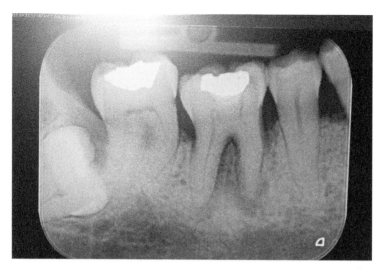

Figure 7.2 Radiograph of periapical abscess at root apices of lower first molar

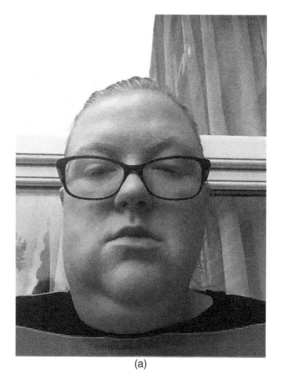

(a)

Figure 7.3 (a) Facial swelling associated with acute abscess of a lower right molar tooth. (b) Intraoral pus-filled swelling

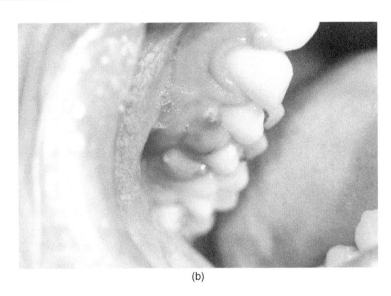

(b)

Figure 7.3 (continued)

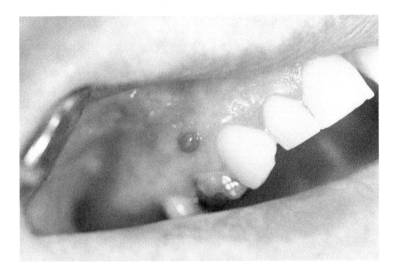

Figure 7.4 'Gum boil' appearance of a chronic infection

DETAILS OF PROCEDURE – PULPECTOMY

Although a dead tooth should be unable to feel pain, many patients are more psychologically comfortable and relaxed during the procedure if a local anaesthetic is administered. The success of the pulpectomy technique depends very much on maintaining a sterile field to prevent contamination of the root canal system with saliva and oral microorganisms, and good moisture control is of paramount importance.

Often the full root canal treatment is carried out in one appointment, but if heavy infection is present or other difficulties occur, then it may be completed in more than one visit.

As well as a full conservation tray of instruments, the additional equipment and materials that may be required to carry out a pulpectomy procedure are shown in Figure 7.5.

TECHNIQUE:

- The dentist, nurse and patient wear personal protective equipment
- Local anaesthetic is administered as required and allowed to take full effect
- The tooth is isolated from the oral cavity, ideally by a rubber dam (see Figure 5.6)
- Access is gained to the pulp chamber and root canal system using a sterile bur in the high-speed hand piece
- All pulpal tissue is removed (extirpated) from the tooth using specialised endodontic barbed broach instruments, which are inserted into each root canal, twisted to engage the soft tissue of the pulp and removed from the tooth, pulling the pulpal tissue with it
- Where infection and necrosis are present, the degenerated pulpal tissue is irrigated from the canals using the irrigation syringe and needle
- The root canal system is enlarged laterally and to the root apex, using endodontic reamers or files, either by hand, with a slow speed hand piece and special files (or reamers), or more usually with specially designed endodontic hand pieces and their own specific files (Figure 7.6)
- The walls of the root canal are also smoothed by the action of the endodontic files to remove any infected tissue and surface irregularities that could harbour microorganisms in the future
- The root canal is irrigated throughout the preparation procedure to remove loose debris, lubricate the area and avoid instrument fracture due to their snatching into the otherwise dry tooth structure and becoming stuck and snapping
- Once the root canal system is satisfactorily cleaned to the root apex and widened sufficiently to allow root filling, the decision is made whether to continue in a one-stage technique or to dress the root canal for a time with disinfecting medicaments to ensure all micro-organisms are eliminated
- Full-length access to the root canal can be confirmed using an apex locator or by taking a periapical radiograph with a file inserted to a known length
- Where digital X-rays are in use, the length of the root canal can be accurately shown using the measuring tool on a previous radiograph of the tooth (Figure 7.7)
- To root fill the canal, it is dried with paper points and then a gutta-percha point smeared with a sealant material is inserted into the previously determined full working length of the root canal
- Similar points are inserted laterally to fully obliterate both the full length and width of the root canal (obturation), or a liquid gutta-percha material can be expressed into the canal before or after the main point is inserted
- This ensures that no spaces remain for microorganisms to linger and recontaminate the root canal in the future
- The tooth is restored to full function and aesthetics, using one of the permanent restorative filling materials available

TOOTH RESTORATION WITH
ENDODONTIC TECHNIQUES

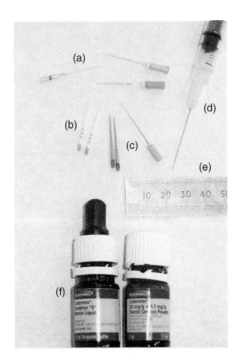

Figure 7.5 Equipment and materials for pulpectomy procedure. (a) Barbed broach and hand files. (b) Paper points. (c) Gutta-percha points and finger spreader. (d) Irrigation syringe and needle. (e) Measuring ruler. (f) Sealing material example

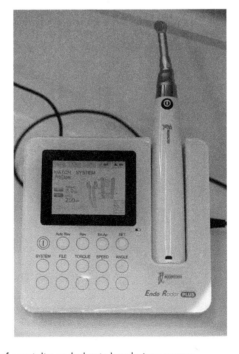

Figure 7.6 Example of specialist endodontic hand piece system

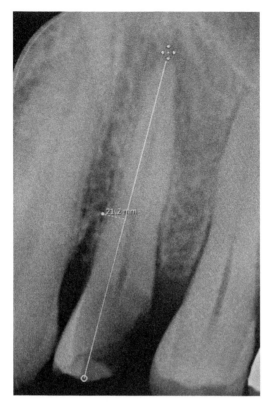

Figure 7.7 Use of measuring tool in digital X-ray system to determine root canal length

AFTERCARE OF ROOT-TREATED TEETH

Although teeth that have undergone pulpectomy are now non-vital (dead), they can still be subject to carious attack if a consistently good standard of oral hygiene is not maintained, or if they are exposed to a diet high in sugars or acids. The patient feels no symptoms of thermal sensitivity or pain in these teeth, and only regular dental examinations will detect the presence of any caries.

If left undiagnosed, the root-treated tooth can become so undermined by caries that it fractures, usually catastrophically at the gingival margin of the tooth. It then requires extensive rebuilding, often involving the insertion of metal or carbon fibre posts into the root canal to anchor and support the rebuilt tooth (Figure 7.8).

Additionally, once their vitality is lost, root-filled teeth can become brittle over time and may then fracture more easily if their structure is not protected soon after the procedure has been completed. Many root-filled teeth are therefore crowned as part of their restoration to full function (see Chapter 6). Similarly, when the endodontic procedure involves the removal of a considerable amount of tooth tissue to gain access to the root canal, a crown is likely to be placed to protect the remaining tooth and help restore it to full function.

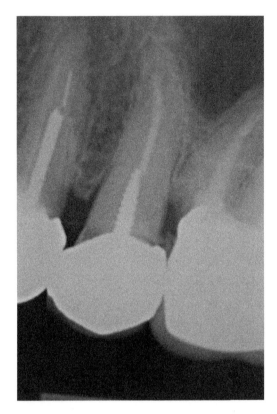

Figure 7.8 Radiograph showing tooth reconstruction involving metal post placement in the second premolar

However, if the tooth fractures catastrophically and is unrestorable, it requires extraction.

BACKGROUND INFORMATION OF PROCEDURE – APICECTOMY

Sometimes, a successfully root-filled tooth can develop an infection around the root apex many years after the initial procedure is carried out, and the associated infected tissues require removal if the tooth is to be saved from extraction. The initial treatment is usually to remove the old root filling, clean the canal system again and re-root fill the tooth. However, if a metal post is present then access to the area of infection is best achieved by a direct surgical technique called an apicectomy. Some other post systems, such as those using carbon fibre materials, can often be successfully removed from the root canal so that re-root filling can be carried out without the need for an apicectomy procedure.

The apicectomy procedure is therefore a third-line treatment in conjunction with conventional root canal therapy, or after the failure of that conventional root canal therapy where access to the root canal system and the apex is prevented by the presence of a permanent post (Figure 7.9).

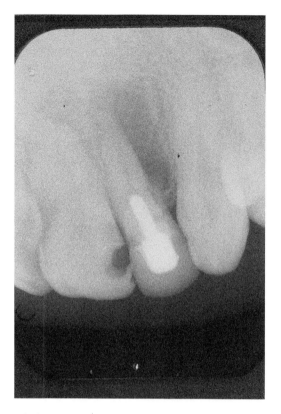

Figure 7.9 Radiograph showing post-restored tooth with recurrent periapical and lateral infection present

DETAILS OF PROCEDURE – APICECTOMY

The procedure is classed as a minor oral surgery technique and is therefore performed under surgical conditions. Although the tooth involved is usually non-vital, local anaesthetic is still required as the oral soft tissues must be cut open to provide access to the affected apex of the tooth root. Once the area of infection and the root apex has been removed from the surgical site, the cut end of the root stump must be resealed to prevent further bacterial access and re-infection and this is often achieved by placing a conventional filling there.

Throughout the procedure, the dental nurse provides adequate moisture control and careful soft tissue retraction, so that good visibility is provided and the patient's oral tissues are protected from possible trauma.

The instruments required for placing a conventional filling are shown in Figure 5.1b, and the available materials are discussed in Chapter 5.

The surgical instruments required to carry out a minor oral surgery procedure such as an apicectomy are shown in Figure 7.10.

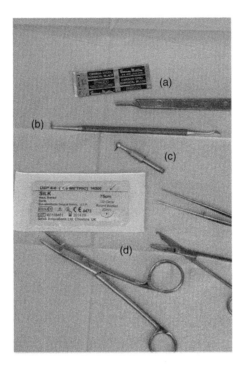

Figure 7.10 Examples of surgical instruments to carry out an apicectomy procedure. (a) Scalpel blade and handle. (b) Instruments to raise the tissue flap off the bone and remove infected soft tissue. (c) Micro-head with bur to prepare root cavity for filling. (d) Suturing equipment

TECHNIQUE:

- The dentist, nurse and patient wear personal protective equipment
- Local anaesthetic is administered and allowed to take full effect
- The surgical site is disinfected using cotton wool rolls soaked in an appropriate solution, such as chlorhexidine
- A soft tissue flap is cut over the affected tooth and adjacent teeth to either side of it using the scalpel instrument and is peeled off the underlying bone to expose the root apex area
- The flap is carefully retracted from the surgical site to allow good visibility and prevent trauma while the rotary instruments are in use
- A small window is cut into the bone so that the affected root apex and its associated infection are visible
- The infected soft tissue is removed and the root apex is cut off from the remaining root structure and removed from the surgical site
- The open end of the root canal that is then visible is prepared using the micro-head and bur and filled using a conventional filling material
- Alternatively, specialised endodontic materials can be used to seal the root canal
- The bony cavity that remains is irrigated with a sterile saline solution to remove any residual debris
- The soft tissue flap is repositioned over the bone and carefully sutured back into place correctly
- The sutures require removal in 7–10 days after the surgery

PATIENT AFTERCARE FOLLOWING MINOR ORAL SURGERY

Bruising, swelling and post-operative pain may all occur after any minor oral surgery procedure has been carried out, as the oral cavity has an extensive nerve and blood supply. Patients are told to expect any combination of these events over the first few post-operative days and are given appropriate advice on the use of pain killers (analgesics) during this period.

A soft diet is usually recommended initially, and a good standard of oral hygiene must be maintained throughout the healing period, but without disturbing the sutures.

Hot saltwater mouthwashes on a regular basis also assist greatly in the healing process, and these can be started the day after surgery and continued until the oral tissues have fully healed. A post-operative radiograph will be taken at a follow-up appointment to ensure that the periapical infection is resolving or already resolved (Figure 7.11).

The patient should be advised to return to the surgery if any of the following events occur:

- Worsening pain, several days after the procedure
- Bleeding from the wound site
- Any discharge from the wound site
- Loss of the sutures so that the wound re-opens
- Extensive swelling, especially within the mouth rather than on the face

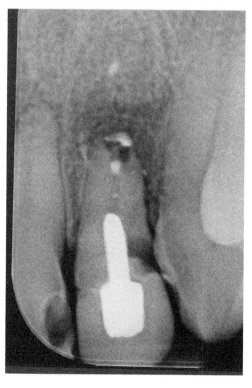

Figure 7.11 Post-operative radiograph showing resolution of previous periapical infection

TOOTH RESTORATION WITH ENDODONTIC TECHNIQUES

Chapter 8

Tooth extraction

Basic Guide to Dental Procedures, Third Edition. Carole Hollins.
© 2024 John Wiley & Sons Ltd. Published 2024 by John Wiley & Sons Ltd.

BACKGROUND INFORMATION OF PROCEDURE – SIMPLE EXTRACTION

A tooth is extracted by loosening it in its bony socket and then pushing it out of the socket, using a variety of dental extraction forceps, elevators, or luxators. To loosen the tooth, there has to be access to the top of the root or roots for the dentist to hold onto with the extraction forceps – the tooth is never held by its crown as this would simply fracture during the procedure.

Alternatively, luxators can be used to sever the periodontal ligament attachment to the tooth and also widen the bony socket so that the tooth is loosened. It is then pushed out of the socket as the instrument is pushed apically.

Physical strength is less of an issue in successful tooth extraction than the skill of the dentist in loosening the tooth.

DETAILS OF PROCEDURE – SIMPLE EXTRACTION

No matter how loose a tooth is, local anaesthetic should always be administered before an extraction procedure. This must be sufficient to numb not just the tooth but all of the surrounding gingiva if the procedure is to be painless for the patient.

The dental nurse provides good moisture control in the oral cavity using high-speed suction, as well as providing head support to stabilise the patient and assist the dentist during the procedure.

Extraction forceps are designed to be used on certain teeth only, rather than universally, and there are therefore many patterns of design available, depending on the tooth to be extracted. Those required to extract a tooth are shown in Figure 8.1.

Examples of a luxator and various elevators are shown in Figure 8.2.

TECHNIQUE:

- A current radiograph of the tooth is displayed so that the dentist is aware of any root curvatures or the extent of any caries present (Figure 8.3)
- The dentist, nurse and patient wear personal protective equipment
- Local anaesthetic is administered and allowed to take full effect
- The dental chair is angled so that the dentist can apply suitable pressure to the tooth without straining, as tooth extraction requires some physical exertion
- The dental nurse may need to support the patient's head firmly but comfortably to prevent rocking movements, as these waste the physical effort of the dentist during the extraction
- The dentist uses extraction forceps, luxators and/or elevators to gradually loosen the periodontal attachment of the tooth root to the bony socket walls
- High-speed suction is used by the dental nurse to remove any blood and keep the operative field visually clear for the dentist
- The tooth is firmly held by the forceps and removed from the oral cavity as the extraction is completed

(continued)

TOOTH EXTRACTION

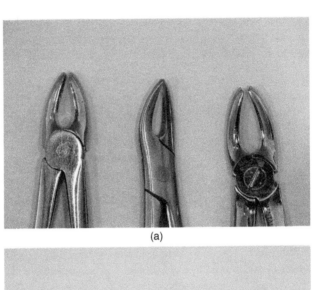

(a)

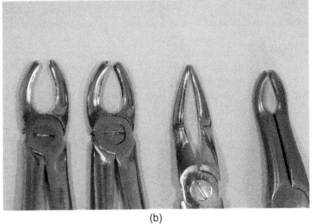

(b)

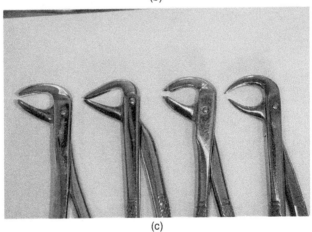

(c)

Figure 8.1 Examples of extraction forceps. (a) Upper anterior and premolar teeth/roots. (b) Upper molar teeth/roots. (c) Lower teeth and roots

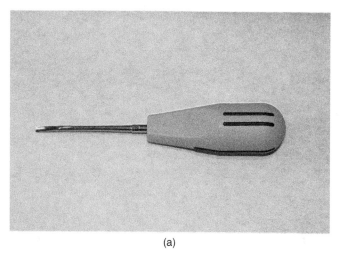

(a)

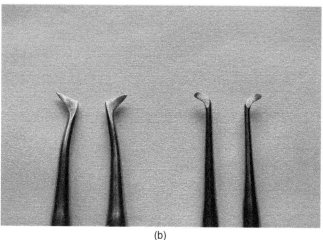

(b)

Figure 8.2 Examples of other extraction instruments. (a) Luxator. (b) Elevators

TECHNIQUE: (*Continued*)

- A bite pack is placed over the socket, and the patient is instructed to bite down hard onto it to achieve haemostasis
- The tooth is inspected to ensure that it has been extracted whole, and that no fractured root fragments remain in the socket
- The socket is inspected once bleeding has stopped to ensure that no bony fractures to the socket wall have occurred – any loose sequestra are removed
- Full written post-operative instructions (Figure 8.4) are gone through verbally and given to the patient, so that the patient is aware of how to keep the area clean and to ensure the socket heals uneventfully

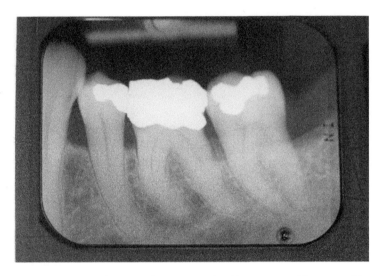

Figure 8.3 Pre-extraction radiograph showing considerable curvature of front root of lower molar tooth

What to do after a tooth extraction

Most patients heal quickly and uneventfully after having a tooth extraction. Problems will occur if the blood clot which forms in the tooth socket is dislodged, or if the socket is not kept clean during the healing period.

To avoid dislodging the blood clot you must not do any of the following for the rest of the day:

- Take any exercise or carry out any manual work
- Drink any alcohol or hot drinks
- Smoke
- Rinse your mouth out

Do not eat or drink anything until the anaesthetic has worn off, as you may bite, burn, or scald yourself. Once the anaesthetic has worn off, you may eat cold or warm foods (not hot) but keep the food away from the tooth socket so that the blood clot is not disturbed. Cold or lukewarm drinks may also be taken, but do not rinse them around your mouth before swallowing.

To keep the socket clean you must do the following:

- Use hot salt water mouthwashes after each meal, from the day after the extraction
- Use a teaspoon of salt per glass of water, and use the glassful each time
- Do these for a minimum of three days after the extraction, or as instructed by the dentist
- Do not use other mouthwashes for at least three days
- Avoid touching the socket with your fingers or other objects, as infection may be introduced
- All other teeth must be brushed as usual, but take care around the extraction site

Figure 8.4 Example of written post-operative instruction leaflet

TOOTH EXTRACTION

Pain relief

Normal pain killers (such as those used for a headache) can be taken if necessary after the extraction, but do not exceed the stated dose, and do not use aspirin-based pain killers. Aspirin thins the blood by reducing clotting, and its use will allow bleeding to occur. If pain begins several days after the extraction, contact the surgery for advice.

If bleeding occurs after several hours you must do the following:

- Stop whatever caused the bleeding to resume (exercise, rinsing, and so on)
- Place a dampened cotton cloth over the socket and bite firmly on it for at least thirty minutes, and repeat this action up to three times
- Contact the surgery for advice if the bleeding continues after this timeaa

Figure 8.4 (*continued*)

PATIENT AFTERCARE FOLLOWING A SIMPLE EXTRACTION

It is particularly important after an extraction for the patient to follow the post-operative advice that is given by the oral health team – that is why the instructions are given both verbally at the surgery (so the patient can ask any questions) and also in a written format (so that they can be read again at home and referred to by the patient as required).

Failure to follow the post-operative instructions is likely to result in a problem developing for the patient, usually a painful one. The instructions given are detailed as follows, with an explanation of their relevance and importance:

- Bite on the bite pack for a minimum of 15 minutes – this applies pressure to the torn blood vessels in the extraction site and assists in their constriction and in the control of haemorrhage from the wound
- Do nothing to encourage the wound to start bleeding again – therefore the patient should refrain from exercise, alcohol, hot drinks, mouth rinsing and touching the wound for the next 24 h
- Hot saltwater mouthwashes – these start the day after the extraction and should be carried out at least 3 times daily for a minimum of 3 days, to help clean the wound and encourage healing
- Refrain from smoking – there is an increased risk of developing a post-operative infection in the wound if the patient smokes while the socket is still raw
- Eating – the patient can eat once the local anaesthetic has worn off but must avoid the extraction site and take warm, bland foods only, so that the tissues are not irritated during healing
- Analgesics – the patient can take pain killers if necessary but must not exceed the correct dose and must avoid aspirin-based products as these act as anticoagulants and allow bleeding to recur
- Problems – if there is severe pain, swelling or recurrent bleeding, contact the surgery for emergency advice, and treatment where necessary

TOOTH EXTRACTION

BACKGROUND INFORMATION OF PROCEDURE – SURGICAL EXTRACTIONS

When a tooth has decayed such that caries undermines the crown or extends into the roots, it is likely to fracture during a simple extraction attempt (Figure 8.5). Similarly, a heavily filled tooth is weak to the forces applied during extraction and may also fracture and disintegrate during the procedure.

Some teeth, especially multi-rooted posterior ones, have curved roots that make simple extraction difficult, as attempts to elevate it from the socket in one direction often lock the curved root in place (see Figure 8.3).

Partially erupted teeth (and obviously unerupted ones) are, by definition, not fully through the gingivae, so access to their roots for extraction purposes is impossible (Figure 8.6).

In all these cases, the dentist resorts to some form of surgical technique to extract the tooth involved, ideally without leaving any pieces in situ.

DETAILS OF PROCEDURE – SURGICAL EXTRACTIONS

When a simple extraction cannot be performed because of curved roots or gross caries, the dentist can often simply section the tooth into its two or three separate roots (hemisection or trisection, respectively) and elevate each one as a single root, without the need for peeling the gingiva from the underlying bone as a full surgical procedure (Figure 8.7).

In all other cases of surgical extraction, some degree of gingival and possibly bone removal is necessary, so again local anaesthetic is required. Specialised surgical

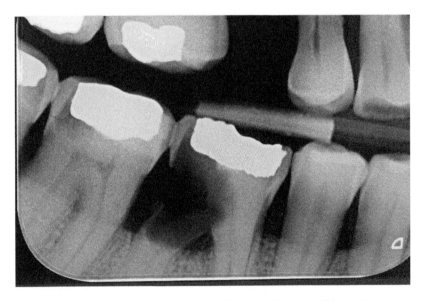

Figure 8.5 Radiograph showing caries extending deep into the crown of the tooth

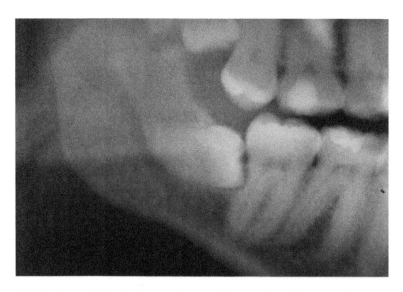

Figure 8.6 Radiograph showing impacted lower wisdom tooth requiring surgical extraction

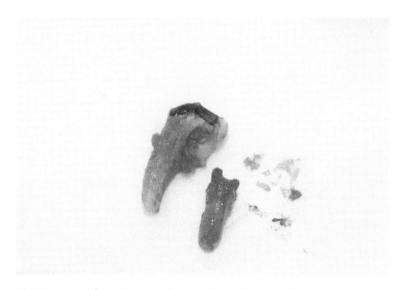

Figure 8.7 Two roots of grossly carious lower molar tooth extracted separately

instruments are employed, and the dental nurse uses high-speed suction and fine surgical tips to maintain moisture control and provide a clear operative field for the dentist.

Examples of the surgical instruments required during a surgical extraction are shown in Figure 8.8.

TOOTH EXTRACTION

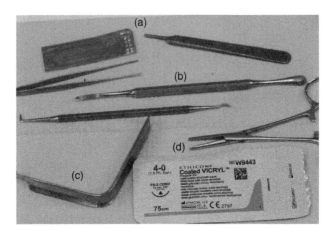

Figure 8.8 Examples of surgical instruments to perform a surgical extraction procedure. (a) Scalpel kit. (b) Flap-raising instruments. (c) Soft tissue retractor. (d) Suturing instruments

TOOTH EXTRACTION

TECHNIQUE:

- A current radiograph of the tooth is placed on display for the dentist's reference
- The dentist, nurse and patient wear personal protective equipment
- Local anaesthetic is administered and allowed to take full effect
- The dental chair is angled so that the dentist and nurse have clear visibility of the tooth without straining, as surgical extractions can take considerable time
- The dentist cuts the surrounding gingiva with a scalpel blade and peels it back from the underlying bone using surgical instruments
- The dental nurse retracts the soft tissues and uses high-speed suction to maintain a clear operative field
- The tooth roots are assessed and bone may be removed to improve access to them, usually using a surgical bur and handpiece with copious irrigation
- Once sufficient bone has been removed, the dentist uses a variety of elevators, luxators and forceps to remove the roots
- Ideally, all the tooth and root pieces are removed, but just occasionally, small but very deeply placed root fragments may remain inaccessible without some considerable bone removal
- A decision may be made to leave these in situ and keep them under observation radiographically, rather than proceed with excessive bone removal that could weaken the jaw itself
- The patient is informed of this decision at the time
- Once the tooth and root removal are completed, the socket is checked for any loose bony sequestrae, which are removed
- A haemostatic sponge may be placed into the socket at this point, to assist with haemostasis but also to provide a physical 'plug', which helps to prevent food debris from contaminating the socket during healing – the sponge is fully resorbable and does not require removal at a later date
- The extracted tooth or root may also have tissue attached to it, such as associated infectious tissue (Figure 8.9) or even a piece of bone that is stuck to the root – the latter may happen particularly with the extraction of upper wisdom teeth (Figure 8.10)

- The gingival tissue flap is sutured back into place to cover the underlying bone and allow healing to occur
- The patient is instructed to clamp onto a bite pack placed over the socket until haemostasis has been achieved
- Full written post-operative instructions are gone through verbally and given to the patient to take home and refer to later as necessary

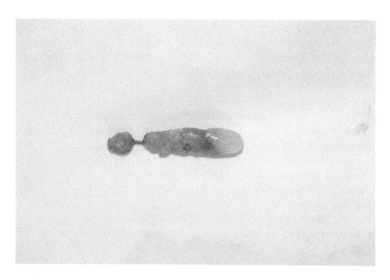

Figure 8.9 Extracted tooth with periapical abscess tissue attached to the root end

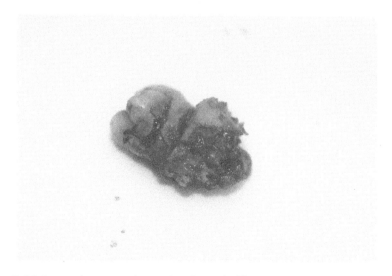

Figure 8.10 Extracted upper wisdom tooth with attached bone present

TOOTH EXTRACTION

PATIENT AFTERCARE FOLLOWING A SURGICAL EXTRACTION

All the instructions relevant to a simple extraction procedure are given for surgical cases too, and the following information is additionally provided to patients undergoing surgical extractions:

- Post-operative pain and swelling – these are likely to occur, as with any surgical procedure, and should be managed with routine pain killers and anti-inflammatories as necessary
- Sutures – the majority of surgical extractions involve the use of sutures to assist the soft tissues to fully heal, and they must not be interfered with by the patient, but require removal by the oral health team after 7–10 days (although some types are available which 'dissolve' over time and therefore do not require removal)
- Post-operative infection – the deeper oral tissues are vulnerable to post-operative infection until the surgical site has healed fully, and the need for the patient to follow the post-operative instructions correctly cannot be over-emphasised
- Arrangements can also be made with the patient to discuss the options for tooth replacement over the following weeks or months and will include:
  o No replacement required
  o Temporary or permanent denture (see Chapter 9)
  o Temporary or permanent bridge (see Chapter 6)
  o Implant (see Chapter 10)
- When implant placement is likely, artificial bone placement may be carried out at the time of the extraction or shortly after, to assist in the success of the implant procedure

TOOTH EXTRACTION

Chapter 9

Tooth replacement with dentures

REASON FOR PROCEDURE

Tooth replacement is necessary for several reasons, the main ones being to provide adequate masticatory function and improve aesthetics. The absence of one or several teeth may also allow overloading of those remaining teeth, so that excessive tooth wear or even tooth fractures occur. When a tooth is missing, those on either side of it can collapse into the space remaining so that the occlusion is altered, or those in the opposite dental arch can over-erupt into the space and cause unnatural wear of the remaining teeth.

Dentures are removable appliances made in several stages in a laboratory, designed to replace just one or several teeth, or a full dental arch in an edentulous patient (those with no natural teeth remaining). Unlike bridges, no tooth preparation is usually required for their construction as long as denture retention is available, and they can be removed from the patient's oral cavity for cleaning as necessary.

They are retained in the mouth by a film of saliva between the oral soft tissues and the denture surface providing suction, as well as by the muscular support of the cheeks, lips and tongue. When the patient has some natural teeth present, additional retention can also be provided by using metal clasps incorporated in the denture design to grip these standing teeth.

The base of the denture can be constructed using a pink or transparent acrylic material, or a very thin skeleton design of chrome–cobalt metal. The latter tends to be more comfortable to wear and more hygienic as less soft tissue is covered but usually requires the additional retention provided by clasps on suitably positioned standing teeth. Alternatively, a thermoplastic acrylic material can be used to construct either a partial or full denture without the need for metal clasps or the reliance on adequate saliva to provide retention in each case. The specialised acrylic looks very similar to conventional acrylic but becomes 'flexible' when immersed in warm water, so that the patient can comfortably insert the denture as it 'bends' around any natural undercuts present in the mouth. Similarly, the warm environment of the oral cavity allows the denture to be removed easily and comfortably from the mouth as required.

The dentures discussed are:

- Full or partial acrylic dentures, including thermoplastic acrylic dentures
- Full or partial chrome dentures
- Immediate replacement dentures

Basic Guide to Dental Procedures, Third Edition. Carole Hollins.
© 2024 John Wiley & Sons Ltd. Published 2024 by John Wiley & Sons Ltd.

BACKGROUND INFORMATION OF PROCEDURE – ACRYLIC DENTURES

Acrylic dentures (Figure 9.1) are the more common type of dentures provided, as they are cheaper and more easily constructed than chrome dentures. They are also more easily adjusted to fit as necessary, as well as being more amenable to relining and tooth addition as the patient's oral cavity alters with time. However, they can fracture during normal usage in patients with heavy bites, as well as if they are inadvertently dropped while out of the mouth.

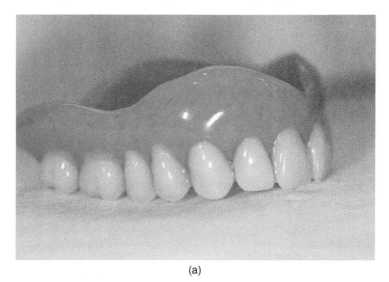

(a)

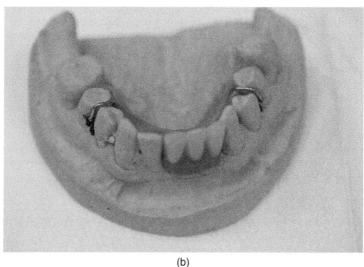

(b)

Figure 9.1 Examples of acrylic dentures. (a) Full upper denture. (b) Partial lower denture with clasps, on model

TOOTH REPLACEMENT WITH DENTURES

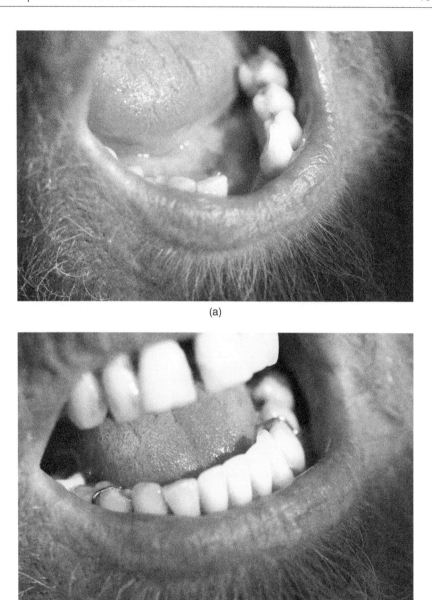

(a)

(b)

Figure 9.2 (a) Appearance without denture in place. (b) Appearance with denture in place

Nonetheless, acrylic dentures fulfil their necessary functions of restoring the patient's occlusion so that adequate mastication is possible, as well as improving their appearance, especially when anterior teeth are missing (Figure 9.2a and b).

Whether one tooth, several teeth or all the dental arch is to be replaced, the construction procedure for an acrylic denture is basically the same.

TOOTH REPLACEMENT WITH DENTURES

DETAILS OF PROCEDURE – ACRYLIC DENTURES

The denture construction normally takes up to five appointments, as each stage has to be sent to a laboratory for the next stage to be constructed. Where a partial denture is being made, the tooth shade is chosen to match that of the remaining standing teeth, but when full dentures are being provided, any shade can be chosen although the dentist tends to advise a natural creamy shade rather than a more unnatural stark white one. However, the final decision of the shade to be used is always that of the patient.

TECHNIQUE:

- The dentist, nurse and patient wear personal protective equipment at each appointment
- The dental chair is kept upright for patient comfort, as well as being the ideal position for the dentist to access the oral cavity for this procedure
- Initial impressions are taken in alginate material and sent to the laboratory for study model casting and the provision of personalised ('special') impression trays to be constructed, as well as wax bite recording rims (Figure 9.3)
- The equipment and materials required for the impression-taking stage are shown in Figure 4.22
- At the next appointment, accurate impressions are taken in one of the elastomeric impression materials available, using the specially constructed impression trays, and the final decision on tooth shade and shape is made by the dentist and the patient
- Occlusal bite recording is carried out using the wax bite rims, so that a partially dentate patient has the same bite with the denture in place as without it, and an edentulous patient can have the bite set at a comfortable position to allow speech and mastication, without the jaws being over-closed or opened too much
- The equipment and materials required for the bite recording stage are shown in Figure 9.4
- Wax bite rims are warmed and stuck together during the bite recording process, and once placed onto the study models, the technician can reproduce the patient's bite accurately
- In complicated cases, the study models may be mounted onto an articulator at the laboratory
- At the next appointment, a waxed-up try-in of the denture is provided, with the teeth set at the previously recorded occlusion and in the shade and shape chosen (Figure 9.5)
- The fit of the denture try-in is assessed for accuracy, although it feels slack to the patient as the wax base warms in the mouth
- The occlusion and aesthetics of the denture try-in are assessed, and any minor adjustments are carried out at the chairside by simply selectively warming the wax bases and adjusting the teeth as necessary
- If any major adjustments are required, the try-in is returned to the laboratory with details of the adjustments required, and a re-try appointment is arranged
- Once the dentist and patient are happy with the try-in, it is returned to the laboratory where a flasking process is carried out to replace the wax base with the permanent acrylic material, as the final construction stage of the denture
- Where a thermoplastic acrylic is to be used, the denture will have been designed to use any natural undercuts around the teeth and bony ridges for retention, and the flasking process is often carried out by a specialist laboratory

TOOTH REPLACEMENT WITH DENTURES

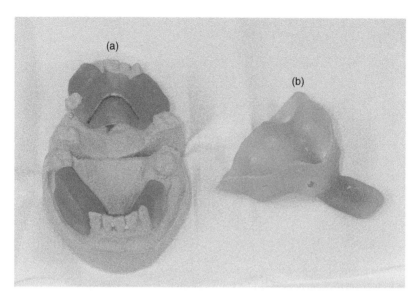

Figure 9.3 Second stage of denture construction. (a) Wax bite rims on models. (b) Special tray

- If metal clasps are being used for additional retention with a conventional acrylic partial denture, they are usually added at this final stage, although some laboratories add them at the try-in stage
- At the final appointment, the completed denture is checked for any sharp edges or specks of excess acrylic on the fitting surface before being tried in the patient's mouth, as these would cause soft tissue trauma with time, if left
- The equipment and materials required for the fitting of the denture are shown in Figure 9.6. The denture is then tried in the patient's mouth and assessed for accuracy of fit, function and aesthetics
- Where a thermoplastic acrylic has been used, the denture must be immersed in warm water to allow the acrylic to become 'flexible' before it can be inserted into the patient's mouth
- Minor occlusal adjustments can be carried out using an acrylic trimming bur and the slow-speed handpiece, so that the patient has an even occlusion around the full dental arch
- Post-operative verbal and written care and cleaning instructions are given to the patient
- Where a thermoplastic acrylic has been used only certain cleaning products are recommended for use, as those suitable for conventional acrylic dentures may damage the specialised acrylic of a thermoplastic denture
- Where a thermoplastic acrylic has been used for denture construction, the patient is reminded that the denture must be made flexible at every insertion by immersing the denture in warm water first

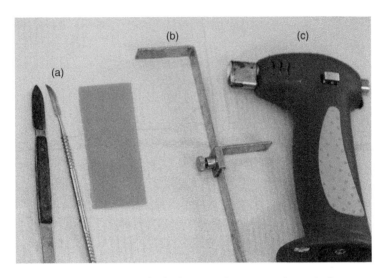

Figure 9.4 Equipment and materials for the bite recording stage. (a) Wax knife, carver and pink wax. (b) Bite gauge. (c) Heat source

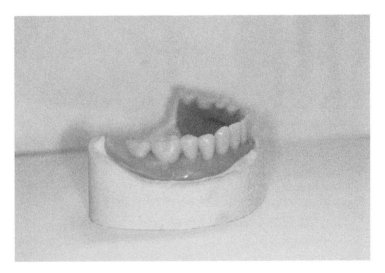

Figure 9.5 Try-in stage of lower full denture, on model

BACKGROUND INFORMATION OF PROCEDURE – CHROME DENTURES

Chrome dentures (Figure 9.7) provide a strong alternative to acrylic in those patients with such a heavy bite that they continually fracture their denture base. As chrome can also be constructed as a relatively thin base compared to acrylic, it is also the material of choice for patients who gag easily while wearing dentures.

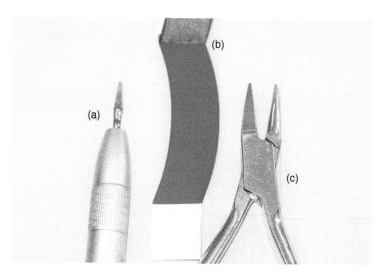

Figure 9.6 Equipment and materials for the fitting stage. (a) Straight hand piece with acrylic trimming bur in place. (b) Articulating paper. (c) Pliers to adjust metal clasps

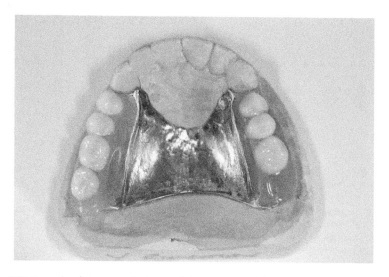

Figure 9.7 Example of chrome–cobalt partial denture on model

As the chrome is so strong, the denture can be designed to have minimal soft tissue coverage and be specifically designed not to cover the gingival margins of the teeth, where plaque accumulates very easily. Consequently, chrome dentures are far more hygienic for the patient, and more tissue-friendly to the gingivae. However, they often require the use of metal clasps around several natural teeth to provide adequate retention while the denture is being worn. In cases where the patient's natural teeth are unsuitably shaped for clasp retention, the dentist can use a routine composite filling material to re-shape the teeth and provide artificial undercuts into which the clasps can engage.

The construction of a chrome partial denture is similar to that of an acrylic one but is less amenable to any inaccuracies of design and fit, as once the rigid chrome–cobalt base has been cast, it cannot be added to or adjusted.

DETAILS OF PROCEDURE – CHROME DENTURES

The denture construction normally takes up to five appointments, with each stage being sent to a laboratory, as with acrylic dentures. Second impressions must be taken using the special trays made from the study models, as these must be accurate for the chrome base to be constructed well and to fit correctly.

TECHNIQUE:

- The dentist, nurse and patient wear personal protective equipment for each appointment
- The dental chair is kept upright for patient comfort and ease of access for the dentist
- Initial impressions are taken in alginate material and sent to the laboratory for casting of study models, construction of special impression trays and wax bite recording rims
- In partially dentate patients, the denture design is developed to make use of all naturally retentive features by placing clasps on suitable undercut teeth, or by using composite material to create artificial undercuts on suitable teeth
- At the next appointment, accurate impressions are taken in the special trays, using one of the many elastomeric impression materials available, such as silicone or polyether
- Occlusal bite recording is carried out using the wax rims, either to maintain the same occlusion or to adjust it accordingly for an edentulous patient
- Again, these can be mounted on an articulator in the laboratory by the technician, if necessary
- The final decision on shade and tooth shape is made by the dentist and the patient
- At the next appointment, the chrome–cobalt base design, including all clasps, is available to try in the patient's mouth for accuracy of fit and design
- Any discrepancies in the metal base require a re-casting to be carried out by the laboratory
- The teeth may also have been added at this stage for a wax try-in or may be added as an additional stage once the metal work has been approved
- The occlusion and aesthetics of the denture are assessed once the tooth try-in is received, and any minor adjustments made at the chairside (Figure 9.8)
- Once the dentist and patient are happy with both the metal and tooth try-in, it is returned to the laboratory for the flasking process to join the metal base to the acrylic gingivae and teeth
- At the final appointment, the completed denture is checked once again for accuracy of fit, function and aesthetics
- Minor occlusal adjustments can be carried out using an acrylic trimming bur and the slow-speed handpiece, but the metal base should need no adjustments
- Post-operative verbal and written care and cleaning instructions are given to the patient, including to avoid bleach-based cleaning products as these are likely to damage the metal components of the denture over time

TOOTH REPLACEMENT WITH DENTURES

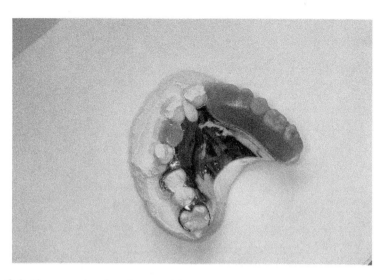

Figure 9.8 Chrome and tooth try-in on model

BACKGROUND INFORMATION OF PROCEDURE – IMMEDIATE REPLACEMENT DENTURES

As their name suggests, immediate replacement dentures are those that are fitted at the time that one or several teeth are extracted. They are usually provided when a patient is to lose one or several anterior teeth and requires the extracted teeth to be replaced at the same time for aesthetics, rather than have visible, unsightly spaces for a while.

Although the aesthetic concerns of the patient are very understandable in these circumstances, it has to be accepted that the resulting denture will not be as accurate a fit as if it had been constructed conventionally – after the tooth extraction and following a suitable period of tissue healing.

Due to the usual event of bone resorption occurring after the extraction, the denture also becomes slack relatively quickly and requires relining or even remaking at some point.

As these alterations are expected to be required, the immediate replacement denture is always made from acrylic, which can be quite easily added to and adjusted.

When significant bone resorption has occurred, usually after 4–6 months, a new denture can be constructed either in acrylic, thermoplastic acrylic, or chrome–cobalt if required.

DETAILS OF PROCEDURE – IMMEDIATE REPLACEMENT DENTURES

The appliance construction follows similar stages to that of a conventional acrylic denture, except that there may be no possibility nor requirement for a try-in if no other teeth are missing except those to be immediately replaced by the denture.

It is imperative that the completed denture is ready for fitting on the day that the patient is due to have the extractions carried out, and this must be checked (as well as that the correct teeth have been incorporated into the denture construction) before the patient's teeth are extracted.

TECHNIQUE:

- The dentist, nurse and patient wear personal protective equipment for each appointment
- The dental chair is kept upright for patient comfort and ease of access for the dentist
- Initial impressions are taken in alginate material and sent to the laboratory for study model casting and possibly for special tray construction
- A special tray may not be necessary if only one tooth is to be immediately replaced, as the completed denture is expected to be less accurate than a conventional one anyway
- Similarly, wax bite rims may also not be necessary if the study models can easily be placed into the correct occlusion without them
- In these simple, one-tooth cases, it is usual to take a shade at the initial impression stage and proceed directly to the final acrylic construction of the denture
- Otherwise, the second accurate impression and occlusal bite recording are carried out at the next appointment, as usual
- The final decision on tooth shade is made by the dentist and the patient, and the technician copies the tooth shapes from the study models
- At the next appointment, a waxed try-in of any teeth already missing is provided, but of course the teeth to be immediately replaced cannot be present at this stage
- The try-in is checked for accuracy of fit, occlusion and aesthetics as far as possible, and any minor adjustments are carried out at the chairside
- Once the try-in and study models are returned to the laboratory for completion of the denture, the technician carefully removes the teeth to be extracted from the model and replaces them with suitable denture teeth, ensuring that the occlusion is not altered during the process
- The flasking process is carried out to replace the wax base with the permanent acrylic of the denture
- At the final appointment, the teeth to be replaced are extracted under local anaesthesia, and once haemostasis has been achieved, the denture is inserted into the patient's mouth
- The aesthetics are checked, and the fit and occlusion are checked as far as possible, bearing in mind the patient is still numb from the local anaesthetic
- Post-operative verbal and written care and cleaning instructions are given to the patient, and a review appointment is provisionally made so that any problems that become apparent once the local anaesthetic has worn off can be corrected

AFTERCARE OF DENTURES

Any type of denture is designed to be a removable appliance, one that the patient can take out of the mouth for cleaning purposes as well as to leave out overnight. Acrylic partial dentures are designed to fit around any standing teeth, and these areas allow plaque to accumulate and cause either localised caries of standing teeth or periodontal disease if the plaque is not removed promptly.

As chrome dentures are usually designed to cover less oral soft tissue, they tend to allow less plaque accumulations to develop. Plaque is still produced in patients with no natural teeth of their own and once mineralised into tartar, deposits can often be seen as a yellow brown crusty layer in the centre of lower full dentures or at the sides of upper full dentures (Figure 9.9). Tartar forms in these areas as they are close to the openings of various salivary glands in the mouth, and saliva provides the minerals for plaque to harden into tartar.

TOOTH REPLACEMENT WITH DENTURES

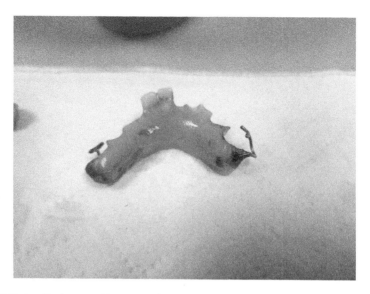

Figure 9.9 Acrylic denture with tartar and stain contamination present

Dentures should be cleaned at least twice daily, using either a specific denture paste or ordinary toothpaste with a toothbrush. They are best cleaned over a bowl of water to avoid breakages if dropped and should be rinsed well before reinserting.

The important surface of the denture to be cleaned is that which covers the oral soft tissues – the roof of the mouth with upper dentures or the bony ridge of the lower jaw with lower dentures. These areas are in contact with the soft tissues whenever the dentures are worn, and any food debris or plaque that is left in these areas allows microorganisms to flourish, in particular a fungus that causes oral thrush and denture stomatitis ('denture sore mouth' – Figure 9.10).

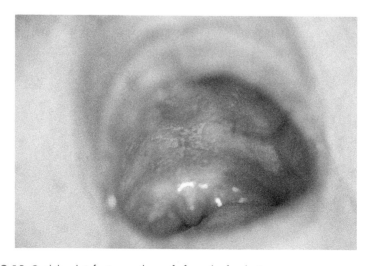

Figure 9.10 Oral thrush infection on the roof of mouth of a denture wearer

TOOTH REPLACEMENT WITH DENTURES

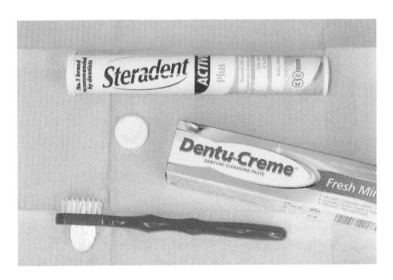

Figure 9.11 Examples of denture cleaning products

Tiny perforations and scratches in the acrylic elements of dentures that occur over time also allow staining to develop, especially with products such as tea, coffee and red wine.

Various denture soaking agents are available for use overnight to assist with cleaning and stain removal (Figure 9.11), but care should be taken with bleach-based ones which are not suitable for chrome dentures, as they cause metal corrosion with time.

TOOTH REPLACEMENT WITH DENTURES

Chapter 10

Tooth replacement with implants

REASON FOR PROCEDURE

Missing teeth can be replaced using bridges, dentures or implants. Each technique has its own advantages and disadvantages, but they are all required for the same reasons – to provide adequate masticatory function and to improve aesthetics.

Implants are the most advanced technique of tooth replacement, although their use has been developing over at least the last 30 years. They involve the surgical placement of a threaded titanium cylinder (implant) into the jawbone where a tooth or teeth are missing, which then has an abutment screwed into its top end to project into the oral cavity. This abutment then forms the attachment for either a crown replacing a single tooth, a bridge retainer replacing several teeth, or an overdenture replacing many if not all the teeth in a dental arch.

The advantages that implants have over other methods of tooth replacement are that they can be used in patients without having to cut into adjacent teeth to construct bridgework, and in patients with very poor retention for conventional dentures. While many dentists are trained and certificated to carry out implants in general practice for straightforward cases, some cases are very complicated and may require specialist input.

These more complicated cases can involve all of the following:

- Oral and/or periodontal surgeon
- Specialist in prosthetics
- Advanced computerised radiographic techniques
- Specialist implant laboratory

The procedure described is for the simple replacement of a single tooth only.

Basic Guide to Dental Procedures, Third Edition. Carole Hollins.
© 2024 John Wiley & Sons Ltd. Published 2024 by John Wiley & Sons Ltd.

BACKGROUND INFORMATION OF PROCEDURE – SINGLE TOOTH IMPLANT

Even when a single tooth is to be replaced, a detailed dental and radiographic assessment of the patient must be carried out by the dentist beforehand. This determines the feasibility of placing the implant and its likelihood of success, as well as the suitability of the patient for the procedure and likelihood of complying with the long-term care of the restoration.

The initial placement of the implant cylinder is a full surgical technique and is usually left in situ for up to 6 months while the jaw bone grows around it to anchor it firmly. Only then is the abutment attached, and the single tooth crown constructed and placed.

During the interim period, the patient is provided with either a temporary denture or a temporary etch retained bridge to replace the missing tooth and sit comfortably over the implant head.

However, more modern techniques have also been developed for use in some cases, whereby the implant cylinder is placed at the time of tooth extraction, and then a single temporary crown is fitted over the top. This can only be done when the replaced tooth is kept free from occlusal loading, so that the bony attachment between implant and jawbone can occur over the following months.

DETAILS OF PROCEDURE – SINGLE TOOTH IMPLANT

Only those dentists who have been suitably trained to provide implants undertake the procedure, as the technique is a specialised field that is not covered by undergraduate training.

Routine radiographs are taken of the area to determine the quality of the surrounding bone available for implant insertion, as well as to determine if the patient has any periodontal disease present. The presence of periodontal disease would usually deem the patient unsuitable for implants, as it indicates an unacceptable level of oral hygiene control or the presence of one or more underlying risk factors that are likely to cause the implant to fail. These risk factors may include certain medical conditions, such as diabetes (often associated with poor wound healing), a family history of periodontal disease, or habits such as tobacco usage. Where the quality of bone is sufficient and no periodontal disease is present, the patient then undergoes a specialised 3-dimensional radiograph (a CBCT scan – see Figure 4.16) to determine the quantity and depth of bone available, so that the required angulation of the implant insertion can be assessed.

Where a patient has insufficient natural bone available in the required surgical area, a technique of 'bone augmentation' can often be used to improve the situation – this involves the insertion of artificial bone products into the area to replace the natural bone that has been lost. In the upper jaw, the natural resorption of jawbone that occurs after posterior teeth have been extracted can result in too little remaining bone being present for implant insertion without the risk of perforating the nasal sinus, and in these cases, a surgical 'sinus lift' procedure can be carried out to overcome this. Once these issues have been discounted or successfully treated, the implant placement procedure can progress.

In a usual single tooth replacement situation, the patient has an anterior tooth already missing and replaced either by a denture or an acid etch retained bridge. The latter is removed intact before the implant placement, and then adjusted as necessary and reattached while the healing process occurs.

Specialist surgical instruments and equipment are required, and the dental nurse provides good moisture control throughout the procedure.

An example of an implant kit containing various items such as bone drills, locators, and various sizes of implant cylinders is shown in Figure 10.1.

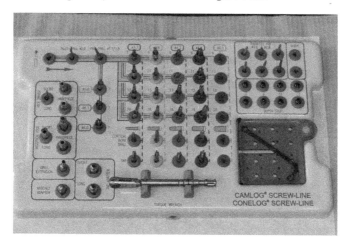

Figure 10.1 Example of implant kit

TECHNIQUE:

- Current radiographs of the implant site are available for reference by the dentist, and the implant dimensions and required angulation of insertion previously determined
- The dentist, nurse and patient wear personal protective equipment at each appointment
- As the implant placement technique is a full surgical procedure, the dentist and nurse wear sterile gowns over their uniforms, as well as sterile hair covers and sterile (surgical grade) gloves (Figure 10.2)
- The patient drapes are also single-use and sterile, rather than the usual clinical (non-sterile) type
- The dental chair is placed at an angle to allow easy and comfortable access for the dentist and nurse, as well as full visibility of the operative site
- Local anaesthetic is administered to all of the surrounding oral soft tissues and allowed to take full effect
- The dentist cuts the surrounding gingiva with a scalpel blade and peels it back from the underlying bone, using surgical instruments (see Figure 7.10a, b, and d)
- The dental nurse carefully retracts the soft tissues and uses high-speed suction to maintain a clear operative field and provides copious irrigation during bone surgery
- The irrigation solution for the procedure is provided as a bag of sterile fluid, which is connected to the specialised handpiece equipment (Figure 10.3)
- The jawbone ridge is flattened at the point where the implant is to be inserted
- A hole is drilled into the jawbone at the correct angulation and to the correct depth, using specialised implant drills (mills)
- The prepared depth is checked using a calibrated depth gauge
- The chosen implant is driven into the jawbone using specialised insert instruments and a surgical hammer, or a specialised slow-speed surgical handpiece, and a radiograph shows its correct positioning (Figure 10.4)
- The implant placement procedure is illustrated in Figure 10.5
- The gingival tissue flaps are repositioned to close the surgical site, with just the implant head projecting through (Figure 10.6)

(continued)

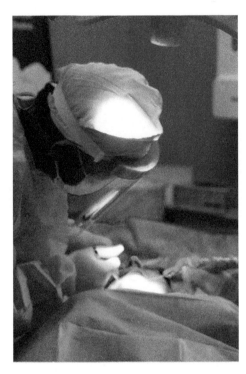

Figure 10.2 Personal protective equipment in use during an implant procedure

TECHNIQUE: (*Continued*)

- If the missing tooth requires replacement during the healing process, the implant head is covered with a plastic cap, and either a temporary denture or a temporary etch retained bridge is placed
- Full verbal and written post-operative instructions are given to the patient
- Following 3 months of healing and the natural attachment of the implant to the surrounding jawbone, the plastic cap is removed and a suitable abutment is screwed into the implant cylinder
- Its shape is that of a conventionally prepared crown core, and its size is dictated by the adjacent tooth positions and the patient's occlusion (Figure 10.7 shows two abutments in place to hold a 3-unit bridge)
- An accurate impression is taken of the abutment(s) and the adjacent teeth, using a silicone or polyether elastomeric material, and an opposing arch impression and occlusion are recorded in the usual way as for a conventional crown or bridge preparation
- The technician constructs the crown or bridge in the laboratory, using the same procedure as for a conventional crown or bridge
- At the final appointment, the crown/bridge is cemented onto the abutment(s) after checking for fit, function and aesthetics and appears not different from a conventional crown/bridge cemented to a tooth or teeth (Figure 10.8)
- Full verbal and written post-operative instructions are given to the patient

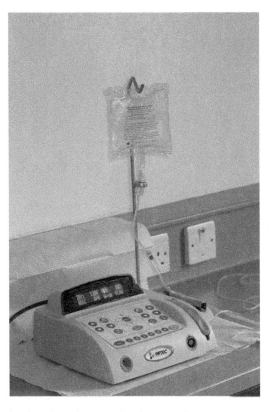

Figure 10.3 Example of implant placement handpiece and irrigation system

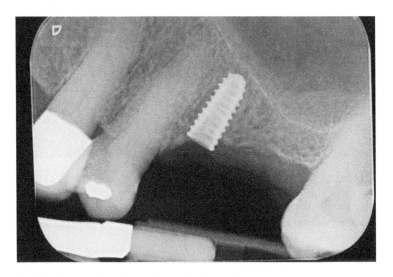

Figure 10.4 Radiograph showing position of implant cylinder

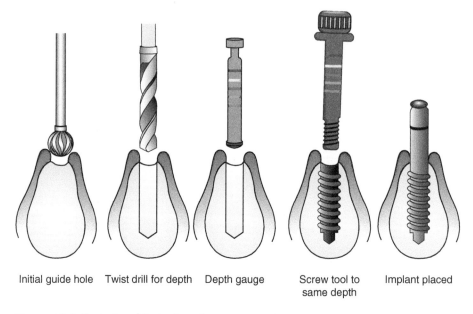

Initial guide hole   Twist drill for depth   Depth gauge   Screw tool to   Implant placed
                                                           same depth

Figure 10.5 Illustration of the implant placement procedure

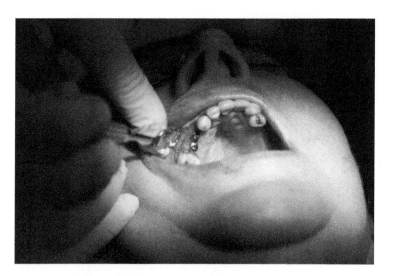

Figure 10.6 Implant heads in place

AFTERCARE OF IMPLANTS

Although the implant cannot be affected by dental caries, it can develop plaque accumulations around it and allow a periodontal infection to occur – correctly referred to as peri-implantitis. Ultimately, this can result in the formation of periodontal pockets around

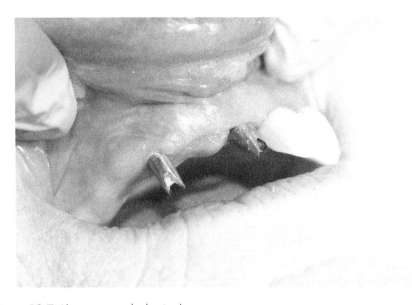

Figure 10.7 Abutments attached to implants

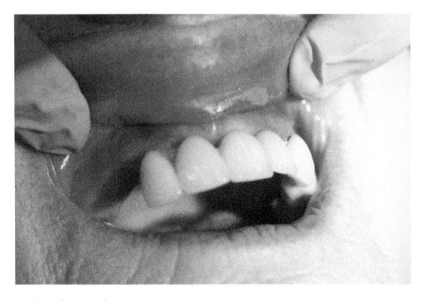

Figure 10.8 Three-unit bridge superstructure in place

the implant, destruction of the bone-implant attachment, and loosening of the implant itself.

As with natural teeth, the prevention of periodontal infection depends on a consistently high standard of oral hygiene being carried out by the patient. This should include correct toothbrushing, the use of interdental cleaning aids around the implant and the use of good-quality toothpaste and mouthwash.

Where bridges are supported by implants, the gingival ridge beneath any areas of missing teeth is cleaned using Superfloss in a similar way to that used for conventional bridges (see Figure 6.7).

Regular dental examinations should be carried out of both the natural teeth and the implant, and regular oral hygiene reinforcement and scaling should be provided for the patient by the dental team as necessary.

TOOTH REPLACEMENT WITH IMPLANTS

Chapter 11

Treatment under conscious sedation

REASON FOR PROCEDURE

Conscious sedation is a technique of anxiety control that uses one or more drugs to induce a state of relaxation in the patient, so that they can undergo a course of dental treatment successfully.

Many patients are fearful of undergoing dental treatment without some form of anxiety control to assist them in doing so; whether they have had a previous 'bad experience', cannot tolerate oral injections or the sound of the drill, have a strong gag reflex that prevents the dental team from providing dental care for the patient, etc.

Whatever the source of their fear of undergoing dental treatment, under conscious sedation the following should be achievable for all patients when successfully sedated:

- Undergo successful local anaesthesia of the treatment area
- Maintain verbal contact with the dental team throughout the procedure
- Remain conscious throughout the procedure so that they are able to understand and respond to commands from the dental team
- Retain the protective reflexes of their airway, so that they can still cough and are not at risk of choking during dental treatment

In addition, the role of the dental nurse in assisting in the treatment of patients who are under conscious sedation is an extended duty (see Chapter 14), with various post-registration qualifications available in the United Kingdom in either one of the techniques given as follows or in both techniques together.

The procedures discussed are:

- Inhalation sedation
- Intravenous sedation using a single drug

Basic Guide to Dental Procedures, Third Edition. Carole Hollins.
© 2024 John Wiley & Sons Ltd. Published 2024 by John Wiley & Sons Ltd.

BACKGROUND INFORMATION OF PROCEDURE – INHALATION SEDATION

This technique involves the patient breathing in a controlled gaseous mixture of nitrous oxide and oxygen through a nose mask, or nasal hood, for the duration of the dental procedure. A nose mask rather than a full-face mask is required so that the oral cavity is accessible for the dental team to carry out treatment unhindered. The technique is suitable for both child and adult patients. Although the gas mixture produces a level of pain relief (analgesia) as well as sedation, it is usually insufficient to carry out dental treatment without the administration of local anaesthetic too.

The equipment required for the delivery of the gases is provided either as a manoeuvrable trolley with all the components present or in dental clinics where many sessions are carried out each week, the gas supplies may be permanently 'plumbed in' and accessed via a delivery unit installed in one or more surgeries (Figure 11.1).

Either way, there are several safety features incorporated into the portable and fixed units to ensure that the patient is kept safe throughout the sedation session and cannot be overdosed with the anaesthetic gases.

- The nitrous oxide cylinder and tubing are always coloured blue
- The medical oxygen cylinder is always coloured black with a white shoulder and the tubing is always coloured white (Figure 11.2a and b)
- The end connections of both tubes cannot be inserted into the wrong port on the delivery machine – they have a pin index system so that only the nitrous oxide tube can be connected to one side of the machine and only the oxygen tube can be connected to the other side of the machine, they are not interchangeable
- The machine is calibrated so that the minimum level of oxygen that can ever be delivered is 30%; therefore, the maximum level of nitrous oxide that can be delivered is 70% although a limiter may be in use that prevents the nitrous oxide flow from exceeding 50%

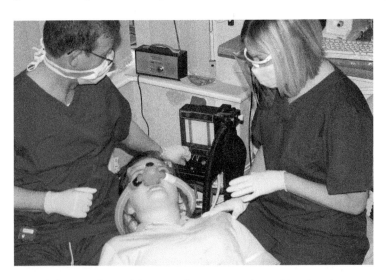

Figure 11.1 Inhalation sedation delivery machine in use with nasal hood in place

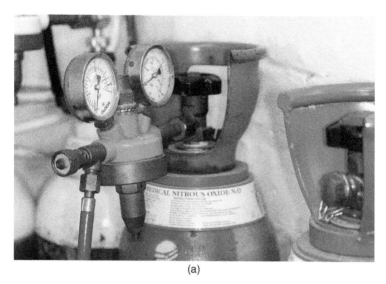

(a)

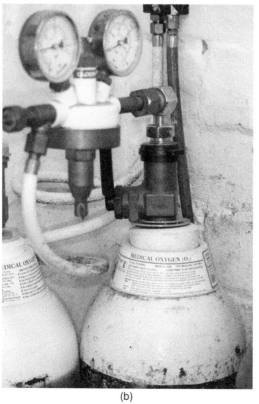

(b)

Figure 11.2 (a) Blue nitrous oxide cylinder and tubing. (b) Black/white oxygen cylinder with white tubing.

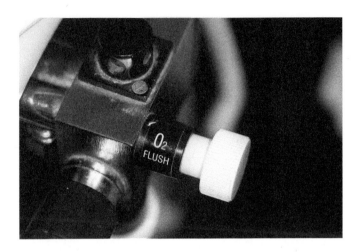

Figure 11.3 Oxygen flush button on delivery unit

- An oxygen flush button enables the nitrous oxide delivery to be stopped immediately, and 100% oxygen to be delivered to the patient in case of emergency (Figure 11.3)
- The nitrous oxide delivery also has an automatic cut-off ability so that if the oxygen flow stops (because the tank is empty, for example), the nitrous oxide flow also stops – the machine will not operate without a minimum oxygen flow of 30%

In addition, and for the safety of the dental team, an active scavenging (air suction) system will forcibly remove the waste nitrous oxide exhaled by the patient from the surgery, so that the team is not exposed to it during the sedation session.

DETAILS OF PROCEDURE – INHALATION SEDATION

At the start of each sedation session and pre-operatively for each patient, the following checks will be carried out on the equipment by the dentist and/or the dental nurse with extended duties;

- Oxygen and nitrous oxide cylinders are switched on and the gases are flowing
- Full spare cylinders of each gas are available
- The reservoir bag is filled with gas and checked for leaks by listening for a gas escape and by squeezing the bag while full to ensure it does not deflate
- The safety features listed previously are checked for their correct functioning, including the active scavenging system
- The flow dial calibrations are checked for accuracy, so when the oxygen is turned to 50%, for example, the nitrous oxide should also show 50%, or 60% and 40%, and so on

Before the patient enters the surgery, they (or their parent/guardian if a child) must confirm that any preoperative instructions have been followed, that a consent form has been signed and that the patient has no condition affecting their ability to breathe through their nose.

TREATMENT UNDER CONSCIOUS SEDATION

TECHNIQUE:

- The dentist, nurse and patient wear personal protective equipment
- The patient is placed supine and a correctly sized nasal hood is fitted over their nose
- 100% oxygen is given initially to enable the patient to familiarise themselves with the sensation and to begin breathing through their nose rather than their mouth
- The dentist adjusts the gas flow gauge to allow an initial 10% nitrous oxide delivery to begin, and then gradually increases this by 5% increments
- The patient is told to expect a pleasant, relaxed feeling as the sedation takes effect – this can be enhanced by the dentist altering the volume, tempo and tone of their voice to introduce a level of hypnosis as they talk to the patient
- Once the patient is relaxed enough to accept local anaesthesia, the treatment session can begin
- Throughout the treatment session, the dental nurse will be visibly and manually monitoring and recording the patient's vital signs (pulse and respiration rate) and noting the maximum % nitrous oxide given over a recorded timeline (Figure 11.4)
- Once treatment is completed, the nitrous oxide is switched off, and 100% oxygen is delivered through the nasal hood for a minimum of 2 minutes to allow the inhaled nitrous oxide to be fully exhaled from the patient's lungs
- The dentist will continue talking to the patient at this time, praising them and giving positive suggestions for future treatment while the patient is still receptive to their voice
- Eventually, the patient is asked to remove the nasal hood, the delivery unit is switched off and the dental chair is gently raised to an upright position
- The patient remains in the chair for a further 10–15 minutes while their full recovery is ensured by the dental team, then they can be discharged from the surgery

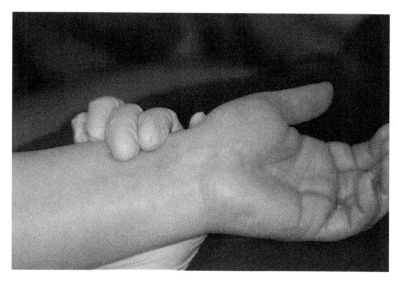

Figure 11.4 Taking the radial pulse manually

TREATMENT UNDER CONSCIOUS SEDATION

The advantages of inhalation sedation over intravenous sedation are as follows:

- Suitable for child patients and adult patients with medical conditions that may prevent them from having intravenous sedation, such as hypertension or heart disease
- Does not involve having to undergo an intravenous procedure
- Patient recovery after sedation occurs within just 15 minutes, as the nitrous oxide is simply exhaled from the lungs without being absorbed by the body
- Electronic monitoring during the procedure is not a compulsory requirement

The disadvantages of inhalation sedation are as follows:

- Cost of the specialised delivery unit and the installation of an active scavenging system
- Nitrous oxide is addictive and overexposure carries significant health risks, so working times must be strictly limited, monitored and adhered to by all dental staff
- Pregnant staff must not be involved in the treatment and care of patients undergoing inhalation sedation

BACKGROUND INFORMATION OF PROCEDURE – INTRAVENOUS SEDATION

This is a technique of conscious sedation for adult patients where a single drug is injected intravenously, using a technique called titration – small increments are injected and the patient's response is assessed after each one until a suitable level of sedation is achieved. In this way, the dentist can deliver the minimum dose required to carry out the dental treatment successfully.

The drug used (Midazolam) not only sedates the patient but also produces amnesia (memory loss) during the procedure and is therefore ideal when prolonged and/or difficult procedures are to be carried out, such as surgical extractions and implant surgery. The technique also gives a more profound level of sedation than that achieved with inhalation sedation.

The drug is carefully injected into a vein on either the back of the hand, the side of the wrist or in the hollow of the elbow, and the cannula used must remain in place until the procedure is over, and the patient is fit to be discharged, in case any emergency drugs need administering. As the drug is injected into the patient rather than just inhaled, the drug and its sedative effects cannot be 'switched off', so the patient requires careful monitoring throughout the sedation session with a specialised machine called a pulse oximeter (Figure 11.5). Most models record the heart rate, blood oxygen level and blood pressure and these readings need to be recorded throughout the session and the records retained – an example of a suitable monitoring sheet is shown in Figure 11.6.

DETAILS OF PROCEDURE – INTRAVENOUS SEDATION

Intravenous sedation is an invasive procedure, the effects of which (as stated previously) cannot just be 'switched off' and the patient expected to recover in time. While under the influence of the sedative, they require careful monitoring by the dental team and then by a suitable adult escort once they have been discharged into their care for the following 12 hours. Written

TREATMENT UNDER CONSCIOUS SEDATION

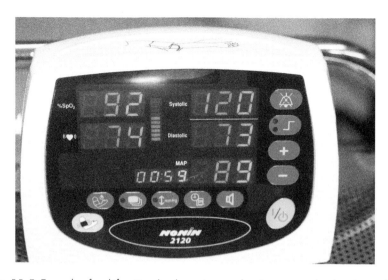

Figure 11.5 Example of multifunctional pulse oximeter, showing oxygen level, pulse and blood pressure readings

preoperative and postoperative instructions must be provided to the patient and the escort, and the written consent of the patient obtained before the day of the proposed procedure. A suitable intravenous sedation consent form with instructions is shown in Figure 11.7.

The sedative drug used may cause a reduction in both the rate and depth of the patient's breathing efforts, and this may be an issue in patients who already have respiratory issues, such as asthmatics, smokers, and patients with chronic lung disorders. Preoperative patient assessment (including a full medical history) by the dentist is therefore key to determining which patients are suitable for intravenous sedation, and which are not. In addition, they must have suitable veins that are ideally visible as well palpable, otherwise the intravenous procedure may be unable to proceed.

On the day of the procedure, the equipment required will be set up ready for use by the dental nurse with extended duties, as follows:

- Multifunctional pulse oximeter, for monitoring purposes
- Oxygen cylinder and nasal cannula, for delivery of supplemental oxygen during the procedure if required
- Medical emergency kit, including defibrillator (AED) and range of airway devices for use if the patient is inadvertently over-sedated or suffers respiratory problems (Figure 11.8)
- Equipment and materials for induction of sedation (Figure 11.9)
  - Tourniquet and alcohol wipe – to raise the vein and cleanse the injection site
  - 5 ml draw-up syringe and needle – to ready the sedation drug for injection
  - Cannula ('Venflon') – to gain access to the vein
  - Sedation drug 'Midazolam' – to achieve the required level of sedation
  - Sedation antidote drug ('Flumazenil') and syringe/needle – to reverse the sedation effect in case of an emergency (such as a fire)
- Mouth props, for use during the procedure to enable the patient's mouth to remain open during treatment (Figure 11.10)

IV SEDATION SESSION RECORD

NAME: **DATE:**

IV DRUG	EXPIRY DATE	BATCH NUMBER	INCREMENTS		TOTAL DOSE
MIDAZOLAM			FIRST	LAST	ml

MH checked:

ASA: I or II

VENOUS ACCESS?	SITE	CANNULA
YES	ACF	23G BUTTERFLY
DIFFICULT	HAND	
NO	WRIST	22G VENFLON

MONITORING TIME	OXYGEN SATURATION	PULSE	BLOOD PRESSURE

RECOVERY SITE	SURGERY ON DENTAL CHAIR		
FIT FOR DISCHARGE	WALK	TALK	LISTEN
POST-SEDATION INSTRUCTIONS	TO ESCORT VERBAL WRITTEN		
TIME OF DISCHARGE			
CLINICIAN NURSE			

© Dr. C. Hollins 2017

Figure 11.6 Example of an intravenous sedation monitoring sheet

INFORMATION FOR PATIENTS UNDERGOING

INTRAVENOUS SEDATION

The technique of sedation by injection in the arm will relax you during your dental treatment. You will not go to sleep. You will be pleasantly drowsy, but able to talk and reply to questions. You may not be able to remember much about the treatment afterwards.

Make sure you advise the dentist of any changes in your medical history, including any medicines you are taking or any visits to your doctor.

The following advice will help you benefit most from this anxiety control technique:

ON THE DAY OF TREATMENT

- Please attend with a responsible adult escort, who is able to take you home and look after you once you have been discharged by the dentist
- Have a light meal a few hours before your appointment; such as toast and a cup of tea – you do not need to be starved for the sedation procedure
- Take any usual medicines at the usual times, unless otherwise directed by the dentist
- Do not drink any alcohol
- Do not wear make-up or nail varnish
- You will be asked to pay for the dental treatment scheduled to be carried out at the appointment before you are sedated – once sedated you will be under the influence of a drug and cannot pay otherwise until the effects have worn off

FOR 12 HOURS FOLLOWING TREATMENT

- Travel home with your escort by car, or a taxi will be arranged – you cannot travel home unescorted or by using public transport
- Stay resting quietly at home while supervised by your escort
- You MUST NOT do any of the following, for your own safety;
    - Use any complex machinery, including a cooker or power tools
    - Drive a motor vehicle – you are under the influence of a drug and are liable to prosecution if caught
    - Return to work that day
    - Sign any legal or business documents, or make any similar important decisions
    - Drink alcohol

HAVING HAD THE SEDATION PROCEDURE EXPLAINED TO ME, I GIVE MY CONSENT TO UNDERTAKE THE DENTAL TREATMENT I REQUIRE (AS SCHEDULED IN MY TREATMENT PLAN) UNDER INTRAVENOUS SEDATION.

I HAVE READ AND UNDERSTOOD THE ABOVE INFORMATION AND AGREE TO FULLY COMPLY WITH THE INSTRUCTIONS GIVEN.

Signed_____   Date_____

Figure 11.7 Example of a written instructions and consent form for intravenous sedation

TREATMENT UNDER CONSCIOUS SEDATION

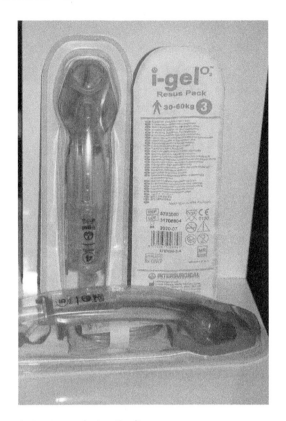

Figure 11.8 Supraglottic airway device: 'I-gel'

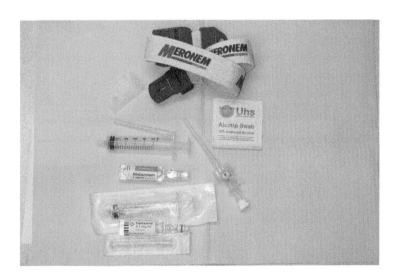

Figure 11.9 Example of intravenous sedation items layout

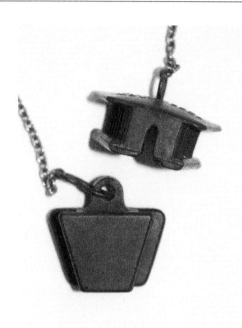

Figure 11.10 Mouth props

TECHNIQUE:

- The dentist, nurse and patient wear personal protective equipment
- The dental chair is angled conveniently for the dentist, depending on which venous site is to be accessed
- Baseline vital signs readings are taken using the pulse oximeter and recorded by the dental nurse – it is normal for the heart rate and blood pressure readings to be higher than expected due to the patient's anxiety (preoperative assessment readings will have determined if a problem existed previously)
- The torniquet is applied to the chosen venous site and the area is cleaned with the alcohol wipe and dried
- The cannula is inserted into the vein, the torniquet is released and the cannula is stabilised with micropore tape or a similar dressing
- The sedative drug is carefully administered using the titration technique, over several minutes and until the patient is suitably sedated using the minimum dose of sedative possible – the concentration, total dose, and time of first and last increments are recorded on the monitoring sheet
- The onset of sedation is indicated by slurred speech and difficulty touching the nose with a fingertip
- A suitable level of sedation is achieved when the eyelids lie halfway closed but the patient still responds to commands from the dental team

(continued)

TECHNIQUE: (Continued)

- Vital signs readings are taken and recorded again – the blood pressure and heart rate should now be at normal levels
- Dental treatment can now commence
- Readings should be taken every 10 minutes or so throughout the procedure and recorded on the monitoring sheet by the dental nurse
- The profound effects of the sedative will begin to wear off around 1 hour after the last increment was given, and the patient will gradually become more alert and communicative – dental treatment should have been completed for this session by then
- The patient continues to be attended to and monitored by the dental nurse until the dentist deems them fit for discharge – usually when they can talk coherently, listen and follow instructions, and walk with little assistance
- The cannula can now be removed and a dressing placed over the injection site
- The amnesic effect of the drug often results in the patient saying or asking the same things over and over again – this wears off over the next hour
- The postoperative instructions are checked with the escort and the patient is discharged into their care
- In particular, the escort and patient are reminded that the latter must not drive, operate machinery, take alcohol or sign legal documents for the next 12 hours

The advantages of intravenous sedation over inhalation sedation are as follows:

- Better access to the oral cavity without a nasal hood in place
- Rapid but controlled onset of sedation
- Very effective degree of amnesia is produced, so no matter how difficult the dental procedure was during the treatment session, the patient is unlikely to remember it – this helps to gradually gain the confidence of the patient to undergo procedures in the future
- No nitrous oxide pollution of the environment and therefore no potential long-term risks to the dental team

The disadvantages of intravenous sedation are as follows:

- Should not be used on children other than by suitably qualified and well-experienced dental staff
- Involves an invasive technique (venepuncture) that may be upsetting to some patients
- Sedation drug requires metabolising and excretion from the body via the liver and kidneys, so some patients (especially the elderly) are not suitable for the technique
- Reduced respiratory rate that can occur may make the technique unsuitable for certain categories of patients and may require others to receive supplemental oxygen throughout the session
- Overdose of the sedation drug may lead to respiratory arrest and require immediate life support to be administered by the dental team, including the use of airways (see Figure 11.8) – all dental staff involved in intravenous sedation delivery must therefore be trained to this level of life support on an annual basis
- Use of the multifunctional pulse oximeter for intravenous sedation is compulsory

TREATMENT UNDER CONSCIOUS SEDATION

Although expensive equipment, potentially dangerous drugs, and advanced training of the dental team are required to provide dental treatment under conscious sedation techniques, their use allows many anxious patients to access dental care who would otherwise be unable to do so. Often, their level of anxiety without treatment access via sedation techniques results in dental neglect, poor oral health and the need for emergency treatment under general anaesthesia – none of which are ideal scenarios. So conscious sedation techniques have a role to play in modern dentistry, with the aim of providing regular dental care to fearful patients while gradually helping them to overcome their anxiety and eventually access treatment in a normal manner.

TREATMENT UNDER CONSCIOUS SEDATION

Chapter 12

Tooth alignment with orthodontic appliances

REASON FOR PROCEDURE

Although a patient's desire for straight teeth is usually based on aesthetics, there are several dental advantages to aligning uneven teeth. Crooked and crowded teeth provide lots of potential areas for plaque to accumulate that would not exist if the dental arch was well aligned. It takes a consistently high standard of oral hygiene for life in these cases to prevent any carious or periodontal damage from occurring with time, as each crooked and crowded tooth area requires individual attention during every toothbrushing session by the patient.

When teeth are severely crowded, they sometimes do not bite together well enough for the patient to chew food efficiently, and in very severe cases where the jaw sizes do not match, the patient may also experience speech difficulties. These severe cases often benefit from a combined treatment approach involving both orthodontics and jaw surgery.

When the bottom jaw bites too far behind its normal position, the upper anterior teeth appear to project forwards quite prominently (proclined), and these upper teeth are vulnerable to trauma or even fracture by being so positioned (Figure 12.1).

Finally, the psychological well-being of the patient should be considered in severe cases, where the malocclusion is responsible for excessively low self-esteem and may be the cause of childhood teasing or even bullying.

The simpler techniques used for tooth alignment are as follows:

- Removable appliances
- Conventional fixed appliances
- Short-term cosmetic fixed appliances for adults
- Non-brace techniques – aligners

Basic Guide to Dental Procedures, Third Edition. Carole Hollins.
© 2024 John Wiley & Sons Ltd. Published 2024 by John Wiley & Sons Ltd.

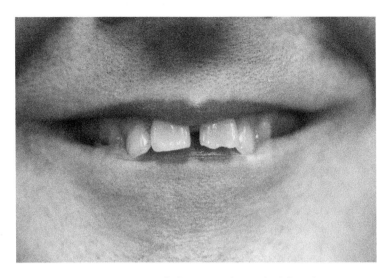

Figure 12.1 Proclined upper incisors with damage evident to the left tooth

BACKGROUND INFORMATION OF PROCEDURE – REMOVABLE APPLIANCES

Removable appliances are made from an acrylic base with metal attachments to provide retention and are therefore similar in construction to that of acrylic dentures. They have additional metal components incorporated as necessary to carry out the required tooth movement to be achieved, and these can be one of a variety of springs, screw devices or adjustable metal bars (Figure 12.2).

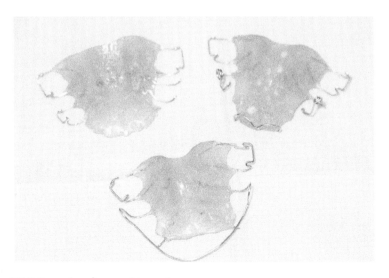

Figure 12.2 Examples of removable appliances

TOOTH ALIGNMENT WITH
ORTHODONTIC APPLIANCES

These components are checked and adjusted by the dentist on a regular basis to affect tooth movement.

Where severe crowding is present in the dental arch, it may be necessary for tooth extraction to be carried out before an appliance is fitted. This creates the space required to reposition the other teeth and align the arch.

The amount of movement possible with a removable appliance is sufficient in many cases to fully correct malaligned teeth, but the force applied is limited by the appliance being removable – if too much force is applied, the brace is not stable in the mouth. It is then that a fixed appliance is required. Indeed, although superseded for most cases by fixed appliances or aligners, there are certain tooth movements that can be quickly and easily achieved with a simple removable appliance alone, especially when used in younger patients while jaw growth is still occurring.

Whichever type of appliance is planned, many new plaque retention areas are created in the patient's oral cavity, and it is imperative that a consistently good standard of oral hygiene and diet control are practiced throughout the course of orthodontic treatment.

Poor oral hygiene is the main factor that prevents many patients from being offered orthodontic treatment, no matter how great their needs are.

DETAILS OF PROCEDURE – REMOVABLE APPLIANCES

The dentist carries out an oral, photographic and radiographic assessment of the patient beforehand and determines the orthodontic treatment required and the appliance necessary to achieve it by taking study model impressions and studying the casts produced. The need for any tooth extractions is decided, and then the full treatment course is put to the patient to decide whether to undergo orthodontic treatment or not. This includes the need for the appliance to be worn at all times except during meals, and the necessity of good diet control and oral hygiene throughout the full course of treatment.

If the patient is amenable to the proposed course of treatment, the removable appliance can be constructed.

TECHNIQUE:

- The dentist, nurse and patient wear personal protective equipment at each appointment
- Alginate impressions are taken of both dental arches for the technician to produce the working casts (see Figure 4.21)
- The written design of the appliance is sent with the impressions to the laboratory
- The patient receives oral hygiene instruction and dietary advice, usually from the dental nurse
- At the next appointment, the new appliance is checked for accuracy of its design and then tried in the patient's mouth
- Once comfortably tight, any metal components involved in tooth movement are activated by the dentist and the treatment commences (Figure 12.3)
- Specific oral hygiene instruction is given for the appliance itself, as well as the wearing details
- At each appointment thereafter, the dentist checks the progress of the tooth movement against the original study casts to ensure it is progressing correctly

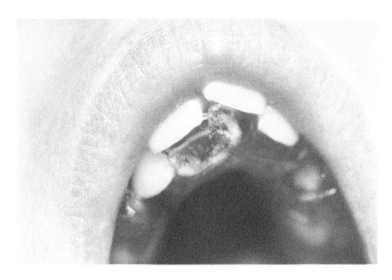

Figure 12.3 Activated spring on the upper right incisor

- Retentive cribs are tightened to ensure the appliance is not loose, and active components are adjusted accordingly
- Various instruments may be required during a removable appliance fit or adjustment procedure
- Once the tooth movement required is achieved, a retainer is provided to hold the teeth in their new positions until they have settled into alignment
- The retainer can either be the deactivated removable appliance itself, or a soft gum shield type, both of which are usually worn at night only but for some considerable time, otherwise the new tooth positions may relapse unless they are locked into the patient's bite following orthodontic treatment

BACKGROUND INFORMATION OF PROCEDURE – CONVENTIONAL FIXED APPLIANCES

As their name suggests, fixed appliances are actually bonded onto the patient's teeth for the duration of the orthodontic treatment. In this way, greater force can be applied and more severely malaligned teeth corrected than can be achieved with removable appliances alone.

However, greater care is needed by the patient during normal day-to-day activities so as not to dislodge any components of the appliance, as the components cannot be removed for meals, cleaning or during sport sessions as a removable appliance can. Similarly, a low sugar and acid diet must be strictly followed, as the number of plaque retentive areas created by a fixed appliance is large, and caries can easily occur around the components if plaque is not removed daily. In the United Kingdom, child patients undergoing orthodontic treatment with fixed appliances are considered 'high risk' for dental caries and should undergo topical fluoride application at the dental practice every 3 months throughout the treatment period too.

TOOTH ALIGNMENT WITH
ORTHODONTIC APPLIANCES

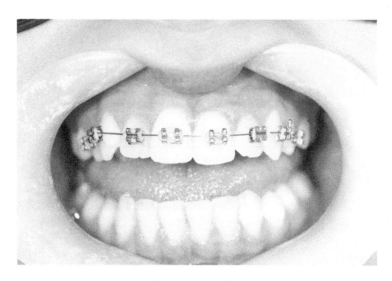

Figure 12.4 Conventional upper fixed appliance in place

Conventional fixed appliances tend to be used in child and teenage patients rather than adults and aim to produce an 'ideal' occlusion in both arches, as well as aligning poorly positioned or crowded teeth.

The fixed appliance consists of individual metal brackets and bands that are harmlessly bonded onto each tooth in exactly the correct position and joined together by tying a continuous arch wire into each component (Figure 12.4). The wire carefully guides the movement of each tooth along it, gradually aligning the dental arch as it does so. The wire is changed on a regular basis by the dentist, using thicker, less flexible ones as the treatment progresses.

As with removable appliances, tooth extraction may have been required to create space in the dental arch first.

DETAILS OF PROCEDURE – FIXED APPLIANCES

The dentist carries out an oral, photographic and radiographic assessment of the patient beforehand and determines the order and progression of the arch wires required, using the initial study casts. The need for any tooth extractions is decided upon and discussed with the patient while presenting the treatment plan. The strict diet and oral hygiene control necessary throughout the course of treatment is also explained, and then the patient decides whether to proceed with the full course of orthodontic treatment or not. If the patient is amenable to the treatment proposed, the fixed appliance can be fitted.

The components of a conventional fixed appliance are shown in Figure 12.5.

The instruments and materials required to bond a conventional fixed appliance are shown in Figure 12.6.

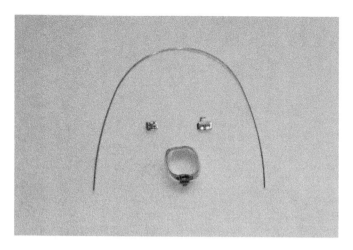

Figure 12.5 Components of a conventional fixed appliance

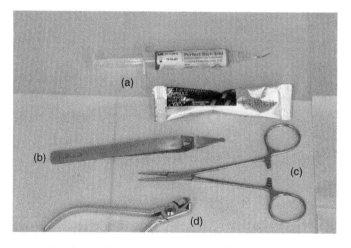

Figure 12.6 Examples of materials and instruments for fixed appliance procedures. (a) Acid etch and bonding material. (b) Bracket holders. (c) Elastic holders. (d) Arch wire cutters

TECHNIQUE:

- The dentist, nurse and patient wear personal protective equipment at each appointment
- The dental chair is placed supine for ease of access, and good moisture control is provided throughout the bonding appointment using low-speed suction and cotton wool rolls
- The decision was made previously with regard to whether just one or both dental arches are to be bonded at the same appointment
- The teeth are blown dry and a spot of acid etch is applied to the centre of the labial surface of each tooth in the dental arch

(continued)

TECHNIQUE: (Continued)

- The etch is washed off and carefully collected using high-speed suction, then the teeth are dried again
- Individual brackets are then bonded one at a time to each tooth, in exactly the correct position and at the correct angulation for each tooth, using a special orthodontic material similar to either composite or glass ionomer materials
- Any bands required are sized on the tooth and then cemented firmly into place using any material that is used for crown cementation
- Once all the tooth attachments are firmly in place, the first arch wire is positioned and tied onto each attachment using special elastic loops
- The first arch wire is usually the thinnest and most flexible available, as it needs to be accurately distorted into each attachment, no matter how malaligned the teeth sit in the dental arch
- The arch wire ends are trimmed to avoid sticking into the patient's soft tissues
- Detailed oral hygiene instructions are given for the thorough cleaning of the appliance, but without dislodging it
- This task may be carried out by a suitably trained dental nurse as an extended duty skill and is discussed in detail in Chapter 14
- At each appointment thereafter, progress is checked against the original study casts to ensure the required tooth movement is proceeding correctly
- The arch wire is replaced as necessary with a gradually thicker and less flexible successor, as the dental arch gradually straightens and the teeth become aligned
- Every 3 months a topical fluoride application is carried out during the normal orthodontic check appointment
- Once the tooth movement required has been achieved, a retainer is constructed for each dental arch to hold the teeth in their new positions until they have settled into alignment
- The retainer may be a soft gum shield type, to be worn at night only, or may be a fixed wire bonded to the backs of the teeth for a firmer method of retention
- In recent years, it has been the norm to provide post-orthodontic tooth retention for life to avoid any relapse, rather than just for a set period of time
- Both arches are then de-bonded, final models and photographs are taken, and the fixed retainers are cemented into place or the removable retainers are given to the patient to wear as instructed
- If necessary, the teeth are scaled and polished to remove any residual plaque or tartar

BACKGROUND INFORMATION OF PROCEDURE – SHORT-TERM COSMETIC FIXED APPLIANCES

For adult patients, the concept of having to wear conventional fixed appliances for up to 2 years to align their teeth is usually enough to dissuade them from undergoing this type of treatment, but very often their only complaint is the appearance of their front teeth alone. Their posterior occlusion (the way their back teeth bite together) has developed and become stable years earlier, so there is often no requirement to adjust the back sections of the dental arches, and consequently, a second type of fixed appliance treatment has been developed for these patients, which has the following advantages over conventional treatment:

- As only the front teeth are to be re-positioned, the treatment time is greatly reduced, and the technique is actually referred to as short-term orthodontics

- In carefully chosen cases, the treatment time is usually between 4 and 9 months, with an average of 6 months (hence the phrase 'six month smiles')
- The back teeth are not moved during the treatment so the occlusion remains stable, as it was before treatment began
- The space required to align the front teeth is provided by careful trimming and adjustment of individual tooth widths as the treatment progresses, and only in rare cases is tooth extraction required
- The components of the fixed appliance used in short-term orthodontics are aesthetically acceptable to adult patients, as they are all tooth coloured

However, not all cases are suitable to be treated with this technique and the dentist chooses those which are appropriate with great care. Children and teenagers are treated using conventional fixed appliance therapy so that the ideal occlusion of the posterior teeth is achieved by the end of the orthodontic treatment.

DETAILS OF PROCEDURE – SHORT-TERM COSMETIC FIXED APPLIANCES

The dentist carries out an oral, photographic and radiographic assessment of the patient beforehand and discusses with the patient the main complaint so that the treatment parameters are determined. Impressions are taken in alginate to provide a set of pre-treatment study models (see Figure 4.21), and a second set of impressions is taken using a more accurate material such as silicone. These are sent to a specialist laboratory where the working models are cast and used to construct the fixed appliance itself.

In the laboratory, the technician carefully places each bracket onto each model tooth in the same way as the dentist does when bonding a conventional fixed appliance in the surgery. Once placed, the brackets are secured into their positions with two warmed sheets of rubbery material that are drawn down over the models under vacuum. When cooled, these sheets are trimmed and split in the midline to produce a quadrant of the appliance for each area of the mouth to be treated: left and right upper arch and/or lower arch (Figure 12.7). These are then returned to the dentist so that they can be bonded to the patient's teeth.

The bonding technique is very similar to that used for conventional fixed appliances, as are the instruments and materials required (see Figure 12.6).

TECHNIQUE:

- The dentist, nurse and patient wear personal protective equipment at each appointment
- The dental chair is placed supine for ease of access, and good moisture control is provided throughout the bonding appointment using low-speed suction, cotton wool rolls and a full mouth soft tissue retractor (see Figure 12.7)
- The teeth in one quadrant are blown dry and a spot of acid etch is applied to the centre of the labial surface of each tooth
- The etch is washed off and carefully collected using high-speed suction and the teeth are dried again

(continued)

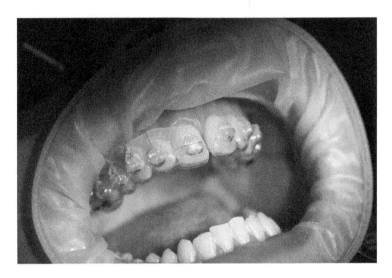

Figure 12.7 Prepared quadrants of short-term upper fixed appliance and full mouth soft tissue retractor in place

TECHNIQUE: (*Continued*)

- A thin layer of adhesive is then painted onto each etched tooth
- Meantime, the dental nurse applies the bonding cement to the brackets in the quadrant that is being bonded
- The tray is then seated onto the quadrant of teeth and the cement is set using a curing light
- Once all four quadrants have been bonded, the double trays are carefully peeled off the teeth, leaving the brackets in their correct positions on each tooth
- Excess cement is carefully removed, and any necessary tooth trimming is carried out to begin creating the space necessary to resolve the tooth crowding
- The arch wire is then tied into each bracket in a similar way to that of conventional fixed appliances
- The bonded upper appliance is shown in Figure 12.8
- In cases where the lower arch brackets interfere with the patient's full bite, small bumps of composite filling material are placed to prop the bite open slightly while the teeth move into better positions – these bumps are then removed once the bite has adjusted and the brackets are safe from being knocked by the upper teeth
- Detailed oral hygiene instructions are given for the thorough cleaning of the appliance, without dislodging it
- At each appointment thereafter, progress is checked against the original study models, any necessary tooth trimming is carried out to allow the crowded teeth to align, and new arch wires are placed, gradually thicker and less flexible as the tooth alignment progresses
- Once the tooth movement required has been achieved, both a fixed retainer and a removable soft gum shield retainer are provided for each arch and are worn for life to prevent relapse of the tooth positions
- Both arches are then de-bonded, final models and photographs are taken, and the fixed retainers are cemented into place
- If necessary, the teeth are scaled and polished to remove any residual plaque or tartar

TOOTH ALIGNMENT WITH
ORTHODONTIC APPLIANCES

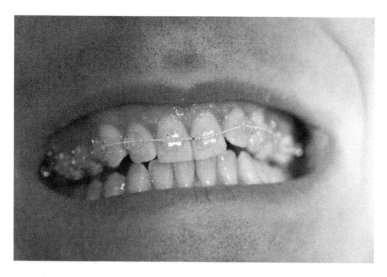

Figure 12.8 Short-term cosmetic upper fixed appliance in place

BACKGROUND INFORMATION OF PROCEDURE – ALIGNERS

For those adult patients who do not wish to wear any form of orthodontic appliance fixed to their teeth, even cosmetic ones, a technique of achieving tooth movement using a series of pre-formed, retainer-like appliances has been developed. These are called 'aligners' (Figure 12.9). In skilled hands, a wide range of tooth movement can be carried out with this technique, without the patients having anything bonded to their teeth, but

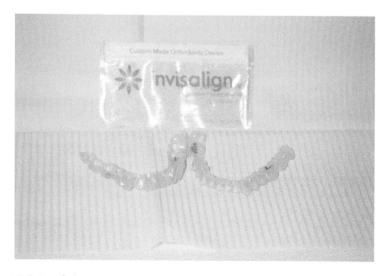

Figure 12.9 Set of aligners

movements such as de-rotation of twisted teeth are particularly difficult to achieve. Nevertheless, aligners are a useful alternative to fixed appliances for suitable adult patients.

DETAILS OF PROCEDURE – ALIGNERS

The dentist carries out an oral, photographic and radiographic assessment of the patient beforehand and discusses the patient's treatment aims to determine the suitability of this type of orthodontic treatment.

Impressions are taken in alginate to provide a set of pre-treatment study models (see Figure 4.21), and a second set of impressions is taken using a more accurate material such as silicone. These second impressions are sent to a specialist laboratory where the working models are cast and used to produce the series of aligners required to straighten the teeth in each arch.

The working models are scanned in three dimensions into a specialised computer programme, which then automatically produces an image of the perfectly aligned arches. The computer then determines the tooth movements required to go from the initial arches to the aligned arches and produces a set of gum shield-like aligners which must be worn in sequence over a set period of time to produce the aligned arch results. These are then sent back to the dentist, who ensures that the patient can insert and remove the first aligner correctly, and so the treatment begins. Some laboratories provide hard copies of the illustrated treatment progression stages for the dentist to refer to so that the required movements of each aligner can be confirmed before moving on to the next aligner in the sequence (Figure 12.10).

Some patients are capable enough to have the full set of aligners handed over at this appointment, knowing the sequence to follow and how long each one must be worn before moving onto the next one, but the majority re-attend to have the aligners fitted sequentially by the dentist.

No special oral hygiene techniques are required as the aligners are removed for cleaning and tooth brushing, but the patients must ensure that they clean their teeth after each meal before re-inserting the current aligner so that food debris is not inadvertently trapped beneath it and does not cause tooth cavities to develop. They must also be reminded not to snack between meals, especially with the aligners still in place – this would allow food debris to become trapped inside the aligner against the teeth, potentially causing areas of tooth decay to develop.

At the end of the treatment, the final aligner may act as the retainer, or silicone impressions are taken and the laboratory produces a separate retainer. The retainer should then be worn 24 hours a day for the first three months, then night times only for a year, and then three nights per week for life.

AFTERCARE OF ORTHODONTIC BRACES

As with acrylic dentures, removable appliances are cleaned with a toothbrush and fluoride toothpaste over a bowl of water after each meal. This is especially important at bedtime as the orthodontic appliance must be worn over night. The patients must also clean their own teeth thoroughly after each meal while the appliance is out, in the usual manner – see Chapter 2.

TOOTH ALIGNMENT WITH ORTHODONTIC APPLIANCES

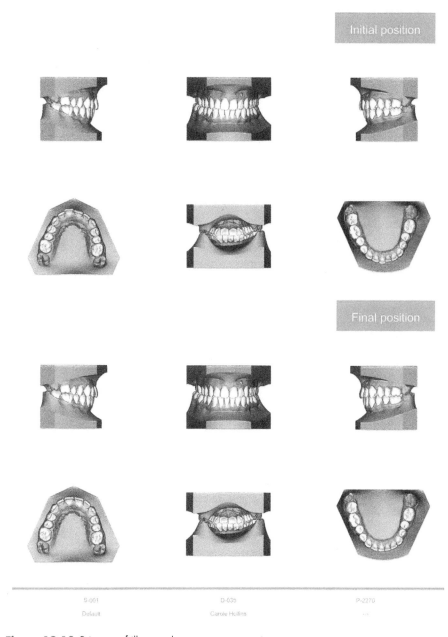

Figure 12.10 Print out of illustrated treatment progression stages

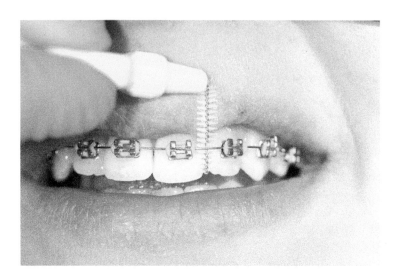

Figure 12.11 Use of interdental brush to clean fixed brace components

Fixed appliances have to be thoroughly cleaned in situ after each meal, using a combination of toothbrush, fluoride toothpaste, and interdental brushes used specifically to clean beneath the arch wire itself (Figure 12.11) – see Chapter 14 for details.

Some good quality electric toothbrushes have special orthodontic heads for use by the patient during the course of orthodontic treatment although more modern electric brushes should also be sufficient without having to change the head.

Patients with removable appliances are advised to store the brace in a rigid container while out of their mouth at mealtimes or during sport sessions to avoid breakages. Fixed appliances can be protected from damage during sport sessions using specially designed shields that fit over them in the mouth. These also prevent soft tissue trauma if the patient inadvertently receives a blow to the mouth; however, contact sports are best avoided during the course of the orthodontic treatment.

If oral hygiene is not sufficiently maintained, or the diet is not correctly controlled, the patient risks developing caries in any tooth, but especially in those teeth in contact with the orthodontic appliance. In fixed appliance and aligner cases, this can result in unsightly cavities on the most visible part of each tooth that will require permanent restorations for life.

Chapter 13

Tooth whitening

REASON FOR PROCEDURE

In an increasingly appearance-conscious society, tooth whitening is becoming a greatly popular treatment for patients to request. In the majority of cases, it is carried out for aesthetic reasons only; however, some patients have unnaturally dark teeth that cause them great embarrassment and low self-esteem. As with some orthodontic patients, the dentist is in a position to improve the quality of those patients' lives by performing a relatively simple and non-invasive technique.

There are a variety of tooth whitening systems available, including over-the-counter products and whitening toothpastes on sale direct to the public. However, patients should be advised that in the United Kingdom, over-the-counter whitening products should, by law, contain lower concentrations of the whitening components than those supplied in products only available from dental practices – the effectiveness of the shop-bought products may therefore be less than anticipated. Also, toothpastes and mouthwashes sold as 'whitening' products often work just by removing stains from the teeth, rather than by changing their intrinsic colour.

When used correctly, licensed products are all perfectly safe and cause no damage whatsoever to the teeth. The alternative dental treatment to achieve whiter teeth is to undergo multiple veneer or crown preparations, and all of the long-term maintenance and care of these restorations that would entail.

The procedures discussed are as follows:

- Home whitening using simple whitening pastes and custom-made trays
- Home whitening using enhanced whitening gels, custom-made trays and post-treatment maintenance products
- In-house power whitening

Basic Guide to Dental Procedures, Third Edition. Carole Hollins.
© 2024 John Wiley & Sons Ltd. Published 2024 by John Wiley & Sons Ltd.

BACKGROUND INFORMATION OF PROCEDURE – SIMPLE HOME TRAY WHITENING

This is a simple technique whereby the patient self-determines the use of the product and the end result achieved. It involves the use of specially constructed trays – similar to thin gum shields or orthodontic retainers – that are worn at home by the patient with the whitening paste within them. Most simple whitening pastes available are advised for use for variable time periods as either daywear or night-wear products, dependent on the concentration of the active ingredients they contain. However, patients must be advised not to exceed the recommended wear times per day of the particular products. Otherwise, the trays can be worn for as many days as the patient decides, and obviously the more usage produces a greater whitening effect, but a noticeable tooth shade improvement normally takes weeks to develop.

As long as the trays fit accurately around the teeth, the treatment course can be repeated as often as the patient wishes and many patients carry out 'top up' sessions to boost the whitening effect, such as before holidays or special events like a wedding. The whitening paste has no effect on any restorations already present though, such as white fillings or crowns, so these may require replacement at a later date if the shade difference is noticeably obvious. Alternatively, where a patient has visible restorations in any teeth to be whitened they can now be replaced beforehand by the dentist, using modern shade-adaptation restorative products. These not only change colour to that of the tooth at the time of initial placement but will also change colour with the tooth as it undergoes the whitening process and therefore will not require removal and replacement afterwards (see Chapter 5).

DETAILS OF PROCEDURE – SIMPLE HOME TRAY WHITENING

Several home whitening products are available to the dental profession (Figure 13.1), but all rely on the use of custom-made trays to hold the paste on the surfaces of the teeth for long enough to have an effect. Other than the provision of the particular whitening

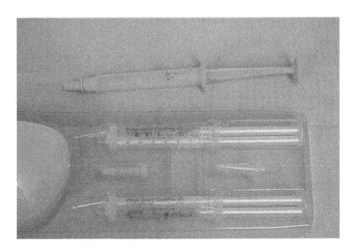

Figure 13.1 Examples of simple home whitening products

TOOTH WHITENING

product and construction of the custom-made trays for each patient, the dentist has little input into the procedure.

TECHNIQUE:

- The dentist, nurse and patient wear personal protective equipment
- The patient will have been examined previously and any necessary dental treatment carried out beforehand, including the replacement of visible restorations with a shade-adapting material in any tooth to be included in the whitening procedure, as necessary
- A simple scale and polish procedure may be carried out if required, to remove any staining or soft debris from the teeth before impressions are taken – gross debris will have been removed at a previous appointment to allow the gums to heal (see Chapter 3)
- Alginate impressions are taken of one or both dental arches, for the working models to be cast
- Using a shade guide provided by the whitening paste manufacturer, the patient's tooth shade is recorded so that the degree of whitening achieved can be quantified
- A photograph may also be taken and kept in the patient's records for future reference
- The cast models are used to construct the customised, vacuum-formed trays for each patient, either in-house or at a laboratory
- The taking of the impressions and the production of the whitening trays are both tasks that can be carried out by a suitably trained dental nurse as extended duty skills – see Chapter 14 for details
- The teeth, which are to be whitened (usually premolar to premolar), have a spacing agent placed over their front surface on the model, which creates a 'well' area in the tray, so that the whitening paste is held in the correct position over each tooth while the tray is being worn (Figure 13.2)
- At the next appointment, the trays are checked for accuracy of fit and then the paste application into the tray is demonstrated to the patient (Figure 13.3)
- Excessive amounts of paste should not be used as this is not only wasteful, but the excess also spills onto the gums and soft tissues and may cause irritation
- Each consignment of whitening paste has patient information details enclosed, and these are explained verbally, then given to the patient for reference, as various products are available for either daytime or nighttime use, with varying concentrations of whitening agent for each (Figure 13.4)
- The patients can request more whitening paste as necessary and can carry out the whitening procedure at home whenever they wish
- Some patients use the technique continually, especially those who smoke and therefore tend to be more susceptible to yellowing or darkening of the teeth
- Others home-whiten sporadically for special events such as holidays, weddings, parties and other special occasions

BACKGROUND INFORMATION OF PROCEDURE – ENHANCED HOME TRAY WHITENING

This newer system of home tray whitening is marketed as producing more reliable whitening results than with the simple home tray whitening techniques, and without the patient having to undergo up to a 2-hour appointment to achieve results similar to those

TOOTH WHITENING

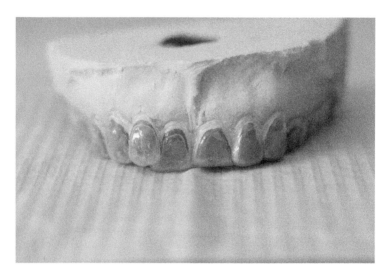

Figure 13.2 Home whitening tray on spaced model

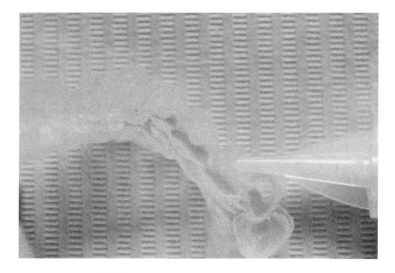

Figure 13.3 Application of whitening agent into tray 'well'

available with the power whitening technique. The results are guaranteed by some manufacturers but rely on the patient following the application regime exactly as instructed by the dentist. It also involves the use of specially constructed trays, as for the previous technique, but the patient must wear them continuously over a 3-week period and with three different whitening gels to be applied in the correct order. If the gels are not worn every day of the three-week treatment period or are not applied in the correct order, the whitening treatment will fail.

TOOTH WHITENING

APPLICATION INSTRUCTIONS

- Floss and brush teeth.
- Twist and pull off clear plastic cap in counterclockwise motion.
- Place mixing nozzle on syringe and secure by twisting in clockwise motion.
- Place <u>small</u> drop of gel in each tooth compartment of tray.

Important: Overloading trays with gel may cause temporary gum irritation, a little gel goes a long way.

- Place tray with gel in mouth. "Bubbling" within tray is normal.
- Remove excess gel with cotton swab or dry toothbrush.
- Remove mixing nozzle from syringe and replace with cap
- for storage after use to ensure ingredients in each side of barrel
- stay separate.
- Rinse trays with cold water. If necessary, use toothbrush to remove residual gel. Place trays in storage case in cool dry place.
- Rinse and brush teeth to remove excess gel.
  Notes: Do not eat, drink or smoke while wearing trays. Area of tooth closest to gums may take longer to lighten than biting edge. It is normal to see dark colors in trays where you have amalgam (silver) fillings. Gel oxidizes surface stains on amalgam fillings.

Figure 13.4 Example of patient instructions booklet

DETAILS OF PROCEDURE – ENHANCED HOME TRAY WHITENING

As with the simple home tray whitening systems, the enhanced techniques also require the construction of custom-made trays for each patient. Once the manufacturer has received the impressions and the patient has been logged onto their website, a personalised patient kit is produced by the manufacturer and sent to the dentist with all the required materials for the whitening procedure.

TECHNIQUE:

- The dentist, nurse and patient wear personal protective equipment for all appointments
- The patient will have been examined previously and any necessary dental treatment carried out beforehand, including the replacement of visible restorations with a shade-adapting material in any tooth to be included in the whitening procedure
- A simple scale and polish procedure may be carried out if required to remove any staining or soft debris from the teeth before impressions are taken – gross debris will have been removed at a previous appointment to allow the gums to heal – see Chapter 3
- An initial kit box from the manufacturer will be assigned to the patient, containing impression trays, impression material and a desensitising tooth 'serum'

(continued)

TOOTH WHITENING

TECHNIQUE: (Continued)

- Alginate impressions are taken of both arches for the working models to be cast, while the serum is given to the patient with instructions to be applied each night at home for the following two weeks while the whitening trays are being constructed
- The serum is used to reduce the risk of tooth sensitivity during the whitening gel applications, as the materials provided with the enhanced home kits are more concentrated and used more intensely than those provided for the simple home tray whitening systems
- A photograph and pre-treatment tooth shade are taken, and the patient is logged onto the whitening manufacturer's website by the practice
- A personalised patient kit is sent to the dentist from the manufacturer, containing the series of whitening gels, the custom-made whitening trays in a personalised tray storage box, and a tube of specialised whitening toothpaste. To ensure, the whitening trays remain in place overnight, their retention can be improved by the dentist applying an attachment to the side of the molar teeth in each arch – simply by bonding a small piece of composite filling material to the tooth surface to help 'lock' the trays in place during normal wear
- The patient then receives the series of whitening gels and strict instructions on their use, as follows:
- Week 1 – 10% whitening gel to be used on all teeth overnight, for the full week
- Week 2 – 16% whitening gel to be used on all teeth overnight, for the full week
- Week 3 – 6% whitening gel to be used on all teeth for 1 hour per day, for the full week
- The whitening gels are applied to the trays in the same way as for those used in the simple home tray whitening technique
- The whitening toothpaste is also given to the patient, with instructions for its use after completing the 3-week whitening gel process as they wish, to maintain the results achieved
- A final appointment is made so that the dentist can check the results, take post-operative photographs and record the tooth shade achieved

BACKGROUND INFORMATION OF PROCEDURE – POWER WHITENING

As the name suggests, this is a whitening technique that provides an instant result for the patient after just one application. It relies on the use of an intense light source to chemically activate the whitening process of the paste after it has been applied to the teeth and must be carried out in a controlled environment at the practice.

As the activated paste is so intense, all the exposed soft tissues of the oral cavity must be protected from contact with it during the procedure to avoid soft tissue irritation or burns. Similarly, the patient's lips should be protected from the light source by being covered with the vitamin soothing oil provided in each patient power whitening kit.

DETAILS OF PROCEDURE – POWER WHITENING

Suitable patients are chosen carefully, as the intense nature of the procedure can cause temporary tooth sensitivity, sometimes intense in nature. This is prevented in the majority of cases by the patient's use of a high-concentration desensitising fluoride toothpaste for

TOOTH WHITENING

several weeks before the whitening procedure is carried out, in a similar way to the use of the desensitising 'serum' used during the enhanced home whitening technique. Also, some medications and even some herbal products can cause the patient to be over-sensitive to the light source used, causing sunburn or sunstroke-like symptoms. Careful pre-operative questioning identifies any likely problems.

Patients who have fixed anterior tooth restorations (veneers, bridges or crowns) are advised that these are likely to require replacement after the whitening procedure, as they are not affected by the whitening process and are likely to contrast with the whitened teeth. Visible anterior fillings can be replaced with a shade-adapting composite material before the whitening procedure is carried out, as the restorations will change shade to that of the whitened teeth during the procedure.

The shade guide is used to determine the pre-treatment tooth shade and should be photographically recorded.

TECHNIQUE:

- The dentist, nurse and patient wear personal protective equipment throughout the procedure, especially orange-tinted safety glasses whenever the light source is in use
- The patient is made comfortable in the dental chair, angled at 45°, as the procedure can take up to 2 hours once started
- The vitamin soothing oil is liberally applied to both the upper and lower lips
- The special lip and tongue retractor is carefully placed in the mouth so that all the oral soft tissues are held away from the teeth
- The inner sides of the lips, cheeks and the surface of the tongue are fully covered with cotton gauze to give full protection and moisture control (Figure 13.5)
- The protective paste ('liquid dam') is carefully run across all the exposed gingival tissues up to the necks of the teeth, then set hard with the curing light so that it provides a light-proof barrier for the underlying tissues (Figure 13.6)
- Each tooth to be whitened is fully coated with the activator liquid
- The whitening paste is carefully and liberally applied to the labial surfaces of all anterior teeth, the components automatically mixing as they are expressed from the delivery tube (Figure 13.7)
- The power light is positioned into the locating fins of the retractor so that it is aimed directly onto the teeth and is then locked in this position for each of the four 15-min cycles of exposure required (Figure 13.8)
- The teeth are sucked clear of the used paste at the end of each cycle then fresh activator and whitening paste are reapplied before the next exposure
- At the end of the procedure, the new tooth shade is recorded and photographed (Figure 13.9), and the soft tissues are checked for any signs of irritation and vitamin soothing balm placed if necessary
- The patient is given full post-operative instructions with regard to avoiding smoking and highly coloured foods and drinks for 48 h, to avoid staining of the teeth, as the teeth are very porous during this initial period
- Any tooth sensitivity is temporary and easily alleviated using a desensitising toothpaste for the next few days

TOOTH WHITENING

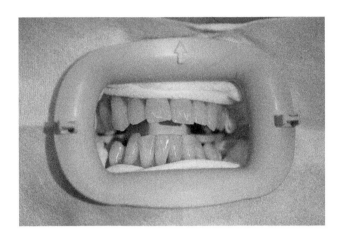

Figure 13.5 Soft tissue retractor and moisture control in place

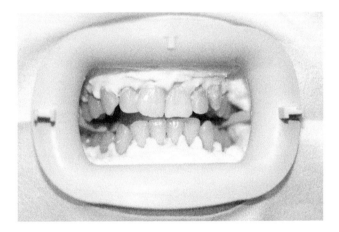

Figure 13.6 Liquid dam full application to lower teeth and during application to upper teeth

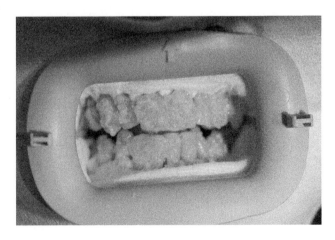

Figure 13.7 Application of the whitening paste to the anterior teeth

TOOTH WHITENING

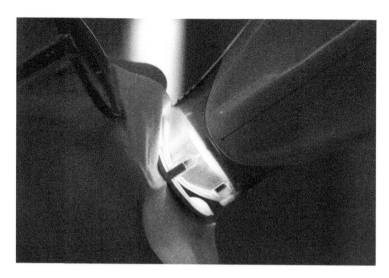

Figure 13.8 Power whitening light in use

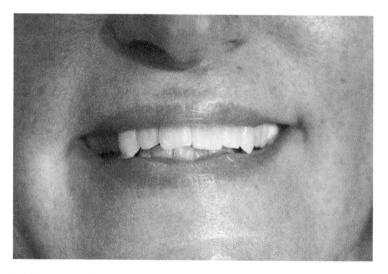

Figure 13.9 End result of patient shown in Figure 13.5 – teeth whitened by six shades

AFTERCARE OF WHITENED TEETH

Any fixed restorations previously present are likely to require replacement, especially after the power whitening technique. Some patients may choose to continue the initial shade improvement achieved with the in-house procedure by using customised trays and home-whitening pastes, and the process is as previously described for the simple home whitening technique.

TOOTH WHITENING

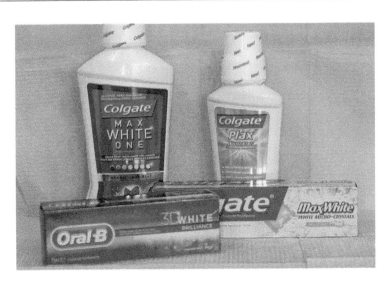

Figure 13.10 Examples of oral healthcare products that assist in tooth surface stain removal

The length of time the whitening effect lasts with no further treatment depends upon the smoking and dietary habits of the patient. In particular, strong tea, coffee and red wine are all notorious for causing tooth staining in any patient, and advice should be given on reducing their consumption for a lasting effect after whitening. The use of one of the many whitening toothpastes and mouthwashes available also helps to maintain the whitening effect when used regularly, by acting to remove surface staining from dietary products (Figure 13.10).

As any tooth whitening technique is non-invasive, no special care and maintenance instructions are necessary, except to carry out a good daily oral hygiene programme.

TOOTH WHITENING

Chapter 14

Extended duties of the dental nurse

REASON FOR INCLUSION

This chapter is relevant in the United Kingdom (UK), where dentists and dental care professionals (including dental nurses) are regulated by the General Dental Council (GDC).

Extended duties are those skills that may be developed by registrants after their initial qualification to enhance the scope of their practice, following appropriate training to a suitable level of competency, and with suitable indemnity insurance in place. It involves undergoing appropriate training in the workplace, which is delivered by a team member who is already trained and competent in the same skills, rather than by attending a formal training course elsewhere. This training is often referred to as being delivered 'in-house', meaning that it has occurred on the workplace premises.

Details of the 'in-house' training must be retained to prove that it has actually been given, and the most suitable format is as a mini hand-out that lists the information that has been passed on to the registrant. Records should be kept of each time that the registrant then carries out the supervised extended duty (including in the patient's records where the skill is used directly on a patient) until the registrant is deemed to be competent – this should also be recorded. Ideally, the workplace can develop and use assessment sheets to provide a record of the supervised tasks, and examples are given for some of the extended duties available to dental nurses in the Appendix. Alternatively, some organisations that run continuing professional development (CPD) courses in the United Kingdom now have suitable online courses available to dental nurses, in topics such as impression taking and fluoride application, for example. Once deemed competent, the registrant's indemnity insurance should be arranged to include cover for extended (or extra) duties, rather than cover just for basic duties.

At all times, all GDC registrants must carry out their duties in accordance with the Council's standards document 'Standards for the Dental Team' and ensure that they never attempt to provide care or carry out tasks that fall outside their scope of practice.

The standards and scope of practice documentation are available to download at www.gdc-uk.org

Basic Guide to Dental Procedures, Third Edition. Carole Hollins.
© 2024 John Wiley & Sons Ltd. Published 2024 by John Wiley & Sons Ltd.

BACKGROUND INFORMATION ON BASIC DUTIES

In the United Kingdom, all dental nurses must be qualified in their basic duties and registered with the GDC to legally work at the chairside, or they must be a student on an approved training course working to gain their basic register-able qualification. The basic duties of a dental nurse are those which they are expected to carry out to provide clinical and other support to registrants and patients and are described as follows:

- Prepare and maintain the clinical environment, including the equipment
  - Set up the surgery area and equipment for a range of dental procedures
  - Maintain the surgery area and equipment between procedures so that it is safe to be re-used for several patients
  - Close down the surgery area and equipment at the end of a work session so that it is safe to be left, and safe to be re-used at a later date
- Carry out infection prevention and control procedures to prevent physical, chemical and microbiological contamination in the surgery or laboratory
  - Carry out full decontamination and sterilisation procedures to prevent cross-infection
  - Dispose of contaminated items by the correct waste segregation category and method
  - Use all accepted methods of preventing contamination of equipment and items in the surgery and laboratory
- Record dental charting and oral tissue assessment carried out by other registrants
  - Tooth charting
  - Periodontal charting
  - Soft tissue assessment
  - Orthodontic and occlusal assessment
- Prepare, mix and handle dental bio-materials
  - Filling materials (temporary and permanent)
  - Impression materials
  - Luting cements
  - All accessory materials
- Provide chairside support to the operator during treatment
  - Readying the patient
  - Having all the relevant equipment, instruments and materials to hand
  - Assisting during the procedure
  - Monitoring the patient throughout the procedure
- Keep full, accurate and contemporaneous patient records
- Prepare equipment, materials and patients for radiography
  - Switch the equipment on
  - Have the correct film packet, cassette, sensor/receptor plate and holder to hand
  - Have the correct patient identified and ready for the radiographic procedure
- Process dental radiographs
  - Use automatic and manual processing equipment, and digital equipment correctly to produce radiographs
  - Maintain automatic and manual processing equipment correctly
  - Replace and dispose of processing chemicals correctly
  - Accurately record quality assurance ratings of radiographs

EXTENDED DUTIES OF THE DENTAL NURSE

- ○ Recognise common exposure, handling and processing faults of radiographs
- Monitor, reassure and support patients
- Give appropriate patient advice
  - ○ Administration advice
  - ○ Basic dental emergency advice
  - ○ Basic treatment advice
  - ○ Basic oral health advice
- Support the patient and their colleagues if there is a medical emergency
  - ○ Recognition of signs and symptoms of various medical emergencies
  - ○ Resuscitation skills, including basic life support and correct use of automatic external defibrillator (AED)
  - ○ Maintain up-to-date medical emergency knowledge and skills
- Make appropriate referrals to other health professionals
  - ○ Refer patients to an appropriate colleague for advice when information required is outside their own knowledge and capabilities

BACKGROUND INFORMATION ON EXTENDED DUTIES

Once the dental nurse has qualified in the basic duties shown previously and becomes a GDC registrant, additional skills that could be developed during appropriate 'in-house' training include the following:

- Further skills in oral health education and oral health promotion (see later)
- Assisting in the treatment of patients who are under conscious sedation (see Chapter 11)
- Further skills in assisting in the treatment of patients with special needs
- Further skills in assisting in the treatment of orthodontic patients (see later)
- Intra- and extra-oral photography (see later)
- Shade taking
- Pouring, casting and trimming study models (see later)
- Tracing cephalographs (see later)

All these skills can be carried out without direct intervention from another registrant once the required level of competence has been achieved. Throughout the working career, the registrant should then attend suitable and verifiable CPD activities in those areas of extended duties which involve direct access to patients (especially the first four duties listed above), so that their knowledge and skills are maintained. Regular monitoring of their competence in the final four duties can be carried out in the workplace by other, suitably trained and knowledgeable colleagues.

Further additional skills can also be developed in the following areas but only when on prescription from another registrant – so a more senior registrant has made the decision that the task is a necessity for a particular patient and has delegated its completion to a suitably trained and competent dental nurse:

- Taking radiographs – specifically, pressing the exposure button when instructed to do so (see later)
- Placing rubber dam
- Measuring and recording plaque indices (see later)

- Removing sutures after the wound has been checked by the dentist (see later)
- Applying topical anaesthetic to the prescription of the dentist
- Taking impressions to the prescription of the dentist or a clinical dental technician (CDT) (see later)
- Constructing occlusal registration rims and special trays
- Constructing mouth guards, bleaching trays and vacuum-formed retainers to the prescription of the dentist (see later)
- Repairing the acrylic component of removable appliances
- Application of fluoride varnish to the prescription of the dentist, or directly as part of a structured dental health programme (see later)

FURTHER SKILLS IN ORAL HEALTH EDUCATION AND ORAL HEALTH PROMOTION

The two main oral diseases – dental caries and periodontal disease – are both caused by an accumulation of plaque, either on the tooth surface or within the gingival crevice or periodontal pockets (when present), respectively. Instruction from the dental team in how to remove this plaque effectively, as well as appropriate dietary advice, is the mainstay of good oral health promotion to prevent dental disease in patients.

Only the most dedicated of patients are likely to maintain a high standard of oral hygiene without any intervention or advice from the dental team, so it is likely that many patients will require regular reinforcement of key oral health messages throughout their time with the practice. As this patient support is often best delivered in one-to-one sessions and can be time consuming, a dental nurse with appropriate training in these extended duties is a huge benefit to the workplace, by allowing the dentist and other dental care professionals to provide treatment to some patients while the dental nurse delivers personal oral health education to others. This system of delegating minor duties appropriately to other colleagues allows the more highly skilled members of the team to concentrate on delivering higher levels of care that only they are qualified to provide. The result is a dental practice that is well led and running efficiently, with a good standard of teamwork in place that enables all team members to work effectively together for the benefit of their patients.

SIMPLE BRUSHING, FLOSSING AND INTERDENTAL CLEANING INSTRUCTIONS

The aim of conventional tooth brushing is to remove plaque from the gingival crevice area around each tooth, and from the labial, buccal, lingual, palatal, and occlusal surfaces of the teeth. Conventional tooth brushing will not clean the interdental areas unless a sonic brush is used, or an electric brush with an interdental adaptation (see Figure 2.17).

Flossing (or the use of dental tape) is ideally used just to dislodge food particles that have become wedged tightly at the contact points between the teeth, while the use of correctly sized interdental brushes is recommended for effective and thorough interdental cleaning of the mesial and distal surfaces of the teeth.

EXTENDED DUTIES OF THE DENTAL NURSE

To ensure that the patient learns from the oral hygiene advice and is willing and able to carry out the instructions given by the dental nurse at home afterwards, the instruction session must achieve all the following:

- Be delivered at a level of understanding suitable for each individual – this involves the use of terminology relevant to each patient, as well as the use of good communication skills; this topic is covered in detail in both text-books dedicated to dental nurse training: 'Levison 12th edition' and 'Level 3 Diploma in Dental Nursing' ('NVQ 3rd edition')
- Be sensible in the advice given – this will involve giving valid reasons for the actions explained and the points made so that the patient can understand why the advice is relevant to them
- Be easily remembered by the patient – this will involve helping the patient to develop a systematic approach to their oral hygiene regime, one that they can follow each day without having to think about it
- Be reinforced appropriately – this will involve the use of relevant patient information leaflets and handouts which the patient can take home and refer to at a later date
- Be recorded in the patient's notes – this allows the advice given to be re-evaluated at a later date by the dental nurse (or other team members) and adjusted accordingly, to ensure that the patient achieves a consistently good level of oral hygiene appropriate to their needs

Tooth brushing

Simply chatting to the patient about tooth brushing techniques will have little effect in improving their skills; they need to be able to see what is being discussed, and ideally to be able to 'have a go' themselves while being advised by the dental nurse (a typical 'tell; show; do' learning experience). A good supply of relevant oral hygiene products and aids is therefore essential to the success of the session (Figure 14.1), as well as a large mirror

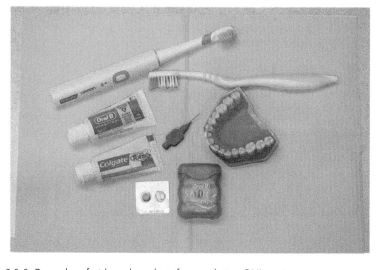

Figure 14.1 Examples of aids and products for use during OHI sessions

EXTENDED DUTIES OF THE DENTAL NURSE

so that they can watch themselves while brushing (so ideally a large wall-mounted mirror). When discussing a child's brushing techniques with a parent, the dental nurse should demonstrate on the child so that the parent learns how to correctly supervise the child's brushing until the child is of an age to carry it out successfully without supervision – usually around 8 years of age (Figure 14.2).

TECHNIQUE:

- Briefly discuss the aims of adequate tooth brushing to the patient, with particular reference to any problems already identified with the current technique (such as missing the lower teeth by keeping the mouth closed, taking too little time and so on)
- Demonstrate the required tooth brushing technique on a dental arch model, so that the patient can see the correct toothbrush manipulation and which areas are to be cleaned
- Allow the patient to 'have a go' at tooth brushing on the model, so that the correct brush angulation and speed and force of brushing are achieved
- Using the model, divide each dental arch into three sections: left side, right side and front, and then divide each section further into actual tooth surfaces
- Refer to these areas in terms the patient can understand – cheek side, tongue side, biting surface and so on
- Ask the patient where they normally start and finish their tooth brushing, and then develop a systematic routine of including each of the eight tooth surface areas in both arches into that regime, so that no surface is missed
- Provide the patient with a waterproof bib and then use a disclosing tablet to expose their plaque retention areas – these can be viewed in the large mirror
- Allow the patient to 'have a go' at brushing the disclosed plaque off their teeth using the new regime that has just been discussed, reinforcing and updating the advice as necessary if they keep missing certain areas
- By the time the disclosed plaque has been fully removed, the patient should have developed a methodical approach of their own to brush all tooth surfaces in their mouth, which they can then repeat at home on a daily basis so that it becomes a subconscious routine
- Effective full mouth brushing should take around 2 minutes, and patients can be advised to use an egg timer or alarm call to help them learn to pace themselves accordingly
- Various Apps are also available to be uploaded to a Smart phone that play familiar tunes and/or show familiar characters carrying out a 2 minutes brushing regime – these are particularly useful in engaging children in effective tooth brushing techniques
- The patient should be instructed not to rinse their mouth after spitting out the excess toothpaste at the end of the brushing session – any toothpaste remaining around the teeth is an important source of topical fluoride which needs to remain in contact with the teeth for some time while it is being incorporated into the tooth enamel
- A small-headed, multi-tufted medium nylon-bristled toothbrush is suitable for the vast majority of patients (Figure 14.3) and is likely to need replacing every 3 months or as soon as the bristles show signs of wear (see Figure 2.8)
- The dentist will recommend a suitable toothpaste for the patient to use, depending on whether they require a good quality fluoride toothpaste or one with additional additives for a particular dental problem (see Figure 2.5)
- Good quality, re-chargeable electric toothbrushes can also be recommended, especially those that use a sonic method of cleaning, as these take the hard work out of the task for the patient (see Figure 2.4)
- The vibratory action of the electric brushes, especially when accidentally caught on other teeth as they are moved around the mouth, does take time and perseverance by the

patient to get used to them – the dental nurse should encourage this perseverance, as the level of cleaning is likely to be far better than that achieved manually for the vast majority of patients

- The patient should also be instructed to clean the teeth over a sink and with the lips closed around the electric toothbrush during use – this limits the amount of 'dribbling' of the toothpaste solution that always occurs with their use and avoids spillages onto clothing
- The benefits of electric toothbrushes should be reinforced to suitable patients whenever necessary:
  - More effective cleaning than manual tooth brushing
  - Sonic effect allows some interdental cleaning to occur
  - Head adaptations allow a variety of uses, including specific interdental cleaning
  - Many have 2 minutes timers incorporated to ensure brushing occurs for long enough
  - Many have 30 seconds beeps to remind the patient to move to the next quadrant; this ensures full mouth cleaning
  - Many have sensors to detect excessive pressure during use; this stops the brush from working briefly and helps teach the patient to use the correct brushing force
  - Heads are interchangeable, so one base unit can be used for several patients within a family, each with their own toothbrush head
  - Heads tend to last longer than manual brushes – often up to 6 months
- A similar demonstration session to that described for manual brushes can be carried out by the dental nurse for patients new to the use of electric tooth brushes

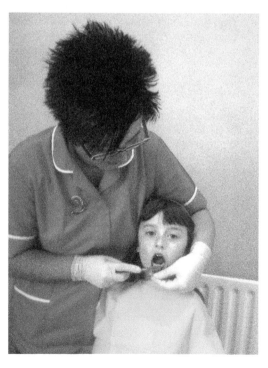

Figure 14.2 Dental nurse demonstrating child tooth brushing techniques

EXTENDED DUTIES OF THE DENTAL NURSE

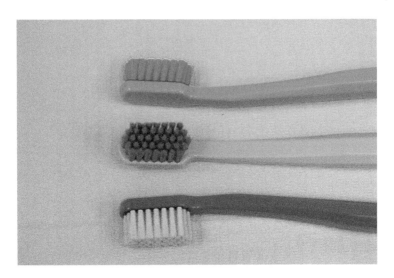

Figure 14.3 Examples of good quality manual toothbrushes

Flossing and interdental cleaning

These skills are required to assist the patient in removing interdental food debris and plaque on a regular basis, where regular tooth brushing alone is ineffective. Again, a clear demonstration of the correct techniques, assisted by good aids and products, is the key to engaging the patients in learning these skills and enabling them to carry them out at home.

TECHNIQUE:

- The technique used to remove debris and clean interdentally will depend to a large extent on the dexterity of the patient, the options being:
  - Use of conventional dental floss or tape (see Figure 2.11)
  - Use of pre-threaded 'flossette' type devices (see Figure 2.10)
  - Use of interdental or interspace brush, depending on the size of the interdental space to be cleaned (Figure 14.4)
  - Use of electric brush adaptations (see Figure 2.17)
- Wood sticks and plastic 'toothpick' equivalents are not recommended for routine interdental use as they are designed more for occasional dislodgement of food particles that have become stuck interdentally – they can also cause soft tissue damage when angled incorrectly during use
- Various interdental irrigation devices, often termed 'water picks' (Figure 14.5), are also available for those patients who struggle especially with interdental cleaning of their back teeth using floss, tape or interdental brushes – although their use can be a little messy, the devices available are effective at washing out the interdental areas and providing a level of irrigation into the subgingival areas too
- A discussion of any prior attempts by the patient to clean interdentally will help to determine the technique that may be suitable for them
- With conventional dental floss and tape, many patients find the use of waxed tape more successful than floss, as the wax allows the material to slide more easily into the interdental

areas without forcing it through and risking cutting into the gums, and the tape then provides a larger surface area for tooth cleaning

- A demonstration is given of how to wrap the floss/tape around the fingers to provide a suitable length, which can be guided into the interdental area and manipulated across the tooth surfaces using the thumbs (see Figure 2.12)
- Once proficient, the patient can be supervised to insert the floss/tape into an interdental area and wrap it around one of the tooth surfaces (mesial or distal), and then use a sawing action to clean the tooth surface as the floss/tape is withdrawn from the area (see Figure 2.13)
- They then unwrap a small section of floss from one finger and wrap it onto the other finger so that a clean section becomes available – this is then guided back into the same interdental area and used to clean the opposing tooth surface in the same way
- Patients who struggle with this technique for their posterior teeth can be instructed in the use of 'flossette' type devices in the same way to clean these interdental areas (see Figure 2.10)
- It may take several devices to clean the interdental areas fully, as the floss/tape is secured in the prongs and cannot be changed once soiled – the patient should be discouraged from continuing to use a heavily soiled 'flossette' as they are merely transferring plaque and food debris from one interdental area to another, rather than cleaning the tooth surfaces
- A far more effective way of cleaning interdentally is with the use of suitably sized interdental brushes and their use should be encouraged in most patients
- Determine the size necessary for the patient (see Figure 2.15) and demonstrate how the brush end can be angled to access posterior interdental areas more easily (Figure 14.6)
- Allow the patient to 'have a go' at inserting the interdental brush in various areas of their mouth, and then use a brushing and twisting action to clean the tooth surfaces before withdrawing it (see Figure 2.16)
- Some patients may need to use different-sized interdental brushes to clean the whole dentition; especially where they have areas of tooth crowding that require small brushes, or spaced teeth that require wider brushes to clean effectively
- The brush should also be used with a smear of toothpaste applied, so that fluoride and cleaning agents in the toothpaste are also introduced into the interdental areas
- Large interdental brushes or even interspace brushes are more suitable where large gaps are present between teeth, such as where a tooth is missing from the arch
- The brushes can be rinsed clean and re-used but must be discarded when the bristles show signs of wear
- For those patients who routinely use an electric brush to carry out their oral hygiene regime, or those who are suitable to be advised to do so, various interdental and interspace head adaptors are available with good quality varieties, which are used to simulate the manual techniques described

DIET ADVICE

Regular and efficient plaque removal will help prevent caries and gingival and periodontal problems from developing, but the incidence of caries is also greatly influenced by the patient's diet. A diet containing regular free sugars (previously called non-milk extrinsic sugars) and dietary acids will always have the potential to allow caries to occur, no matter how effective the oral hygiene regime is.

EXTENDED DUTIES OF THE DENTAL NURSE

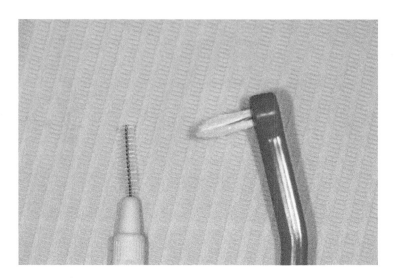

Figure 14.4 Interdental and interspace brushes

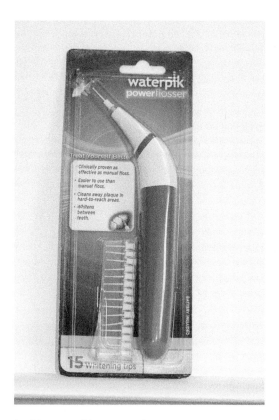

Figure 14.5 Example of 'water pick' irrigation device

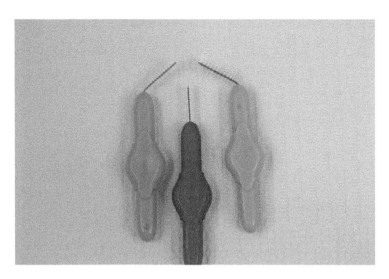

Figure 14.6 Interdental brushes showing angulation for easier use posteriorly

The vast majority of patients are aware of the potential for obvious foods and drinks to cause caries, such as chocolates, cakes, carbonated drinks, biscuits and so on. What many are unaware of are the 'hidden sugars' in many foods and drinks, the role that acidic products have in causing caries and tooth erosion, and the importance of frequency and timing of the consumption of these products in the development of caries. Dietary advice should be geared around these areas.

To give effective diet advice, the patient's dietary contents and habits first need to be known, and the most effective way of discovering this information is to have the patient complete a diet sheet like the one shown as follows. The aim is to have an accurate record of the following points on a daily basis:

- What food and drink are consumed
- When they are consumed throughout a 24-hour period
- When any oral hygiene procedures are carried out during the same time cycle
- What variations there are from day to day, with both the products consumed and the oral hygiene procedures undertaken

To be effective, the patient has to be totally honest – and this must be emphasised before proceeding with a dietary recording and analysis, otherwise there is little point in continuing. The desire to help the patient avoid future restorative dental treatment (and its cost) and to maintain a healthy smile should be stressed from the outset by the dental nurse.

A selection of packaging from various food and drink products containing hidden sugars may be used as 'props' to help convince the patient that the advice is given on a non-judgmental, purely helpful basis by the dental nurse. Again, good communication skills are required if the patient is not to be alienated by the whole procedure.

Once the diet sheet (or sheets if there is a large variation between weekdays and weekends, for example) has been completed and returned to the practice by the patient, it should be carefully analysed to determine the answers to the four questions set previously. The dental nurse may discuss the findings with the dentist or another competent dental care professional, making notes of the relevant points to discuss with the patient. The patient then attends an oral hygiene instruction and promotion session with the dental nurse.

Tuesday	Food or drink	Oral hygiene
6 a.m.	Cereal with sugar, orange juice	—
7 a.m.	—	Tooth brushing, fluoride tooth paste
8 a.m.	—	—
9 a.m.	—	—
10 a.m.	Biscuit, coffee with two sugars	—
11 a.m.	—	—
12 p.m.	Pizza, chocolate muffin, diet coke	—
1 p.m.	—	Chewing gum, not sugar free
2 p.m.	—	—
3 p.m.	Diet coke, chocolate biscuit	—
4 p.m.	—	—
5 p.m.	Cheese and onion crisps	Chewing gum, not sugar free
6 p.m.	—	—
7 p.m.	Chicken burger and chips with side salad, glass of white wine	—
8 p.m.	Glass of white wine	—
9 p.m.	Glass of white wine	Tooth brushing, fluoride toothpaste and general use mouthwash
10 p.m.	—	—
11 p.m.	Glass of diet lemonade	—
12 a.m.	—	—

The information contained in the diet sheet example shown previously, and to be discussed with the patient, is as follows:

Food and drink consumed in this scenario:

- Several obvious sugar and acid episodes
  - Sugar in cereal and in coffee
  - Orange juice and carbonated drinks
  - Biscuits and muffin
  - Wine
- Several hidden sugar episodes:
  - Cereal – even plain examples such as whole wheat cereal and corn flake style products contain sugar
  - Pizza – the tomato paste base contains sugar, as do most tomato sauce or paste products
  - Chewing gum – unless stated as 'sugar free' these products will contain sugar
  - Chicken burger – if additions such as mayonnaise or relish are used

Time of consumption in this scenario:

- The sugar and acid 'hits' occur frequently throughout the day

- This allows potentially harmful levels of food debris and plaque acids to lie in direct contact with tooth surfaces for prolonged periods of time, causing demineralisation

Time of oral hygiene procedures in this scenario:

- Tooth brushing occurs within the hour after breakfast, so some food debris and plaque will be removed
- No other oral hygiene measures occur for the following 14 hours
- This allows all sugars and acids consumed in that time period to potentially cause some caries, especially interdentally where no cleaning technique has been carried out for the whole 24-hour period
- The beneficial effects of the bedtime tooth brushing and mouth washing procedures will be cancelled out by the consumption of the carbonated drink less than 2 hours later
- Also, if the mouth washing is carried out immediately after tooth brushing, the beneficial constituents of the toothpaste will be immediately removed before they have had time to act to protect the tooth enamel
- The carbonated acidic drink then has the following 7–8 hours to lie undisturbed and erode the tooth enamel overnight

Any variations between completed diet sheets for different days can be analysed in a similar manner.

Armed with all this information, the dental nurse can give the necessary dietary advice to the patient in an effort to educate them in reducing the potential harm that their dietary habits may cause. It is unrealistic to expect patients to change their diet completely, and it is highly unlikely that an average diet would avoid all sources of hidden sugars. Consequently, the advice given should focus on reasonable and achievable goals for that particular patient, including the following suggested points.

Food and drink consumed:

- Can healthier alternatives be used, such as
  - Artificial granulated sweetener sprinkled on the cereal and in the coffee
  - Savoury biscuits and cheese (although there is likely to be some hidden sugar content it will be less than for sweet biscuits)
  - Fruit or yogurt instead of crisps (although the yogurt may contain hidden sugar)
  - Limit the carbonated drinks, or have squash drinks instead – even 'diet' drinks are potentially harmful if they are fizzy, because they are still acidic by their carbonated nature
  - Plain water instead of any other overnight drink
- White wine contains less sugar than many other alcoholic drinks such as ciders, sherries and mixers with spirits, but it is still acidic, so the length of drinking time should be monitored by the patient

Time of consumption:

- Frequency?
  - The same foods and drinks consumed in just two or three set meals rather than spread over the 14 hour period will cause less tooth damage, as there are less sugar and acid 'hits' on the teeth

- ○ Can the orange juice be taken before the cereal at breakfast, so that the acid is much reduced before tooth brushing is carried out – the combination of softened enamel from acid exposure and tooth brushing can cause increased enamel loss by erosion
- ○ In particular, the overnight drink of lemonade has the potential to cause massive enamel demineralisation if carried out on a regular basis and should be replaced by plain water

Time of oral hygiene procedures:

- Frequency?
  - ○ Much plaque develops in the mouth overnight, so can the teeth be brushed both before breakfast (to remove that already present) and after breakfast (to remove that developing from the food just consumed) – this will remove the maximum amount of harmful plaque
  - ○ Can a lunchtime oral hygiene procedure be carried out – ideally tooth brushing with fluoride toothpaste, or the use of a good quality mouthwash
  - ○ If not, sugar-free chewing gum will stimulate saliva flow to wash away some debris, and physically pull some particles off the teeth
  - ○ As a last resort, swilling the mouth with plain water after a meal will have some beneficial effect, rather than doing nothing at all
- Procedures?
  - ○ If acids are likely to be consumed on a regular basis, advise on the use of enamel repair products to minimise the erosive effect (Figure 14.7)
  - ○ Avoid brushing immediately after finishing acidic drinks, including alcohol – wait for at least 20 minutes to allow the acids to be neutralised, or use a mouthwash
  - ○ Introduce an interdental cleaning procedure into the regime – bedtime may be ideal as the patient is likely to have more time than in the morning before work
  - ○ If time is an issue, advise the use of a good quality sonic electric toothbrush that will clean interdentally on a regular basis

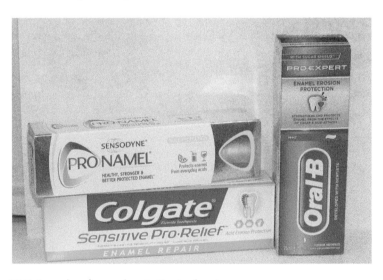

Figure 14.7 Examples of enamel protection toothpastes

○ Use sugar-free chewing gum as a cleaning aid when other procedures are not possible but do not chew gum excessively as this will encourage tooth wear on the biting surfaces of the teeth (attrition)

In summary, any amount of this information and these oral health instruction and promotion techniques can be developed by the dental nurse into personalised oral health education sessions with the patient. The information here covers the basics of oral health instruction and promotion techniques and can be used in total or as a starting point for the development of a suitable training programme.

To be successful in this extended duty, the dental nurse must be adequately trained to become competent in all the following skills:

• Tailor the information to the direct needs of each patient
• Ensure the information is correct and in line with the policies and beliefs of the work place
• Communicate effectively with the patient so that the oral health messages are correctly delivered
• Maintain an up-to-date level of knowledge of the topics likely to be discussed with patients, by carrying out appropriate CPD activities
• Know the limits of one's knowledge and understanding and be willing to ask a senior colleague for advice and direct input when necessary

A post-registration qualification in Oral Health Education is available for dental nurses in the United Kingdom, which trains students to a much greater depth of knowledge in this topic and provides them with a recognised qualification. Further details are available at www.nebdn.org.

APPLICATION OF FLUORIDE VARNISH

Studies have shown that a twice-yearly application of fluoride varnish to both deciduous and adult teeth significantly reduce the caries experience of patients – it is a proven method of preventing dental caries in both adults and children. As the fluoride varnish acts by sealing the dentinal tubules of the tooth (microscopic 'pores' within the tooth that contain nerve endings), it is also a proven method of reducing hypersensitivity to cold in adult patients too. Previously the application technique was only carried out on children, especially where oral hygiene maintenance was an issue and using upper and lower application trays loaded with a thick fluoride gel. Modern techniques are more patient friendly and involve the use of direct, tooth-by-tooth applications using pleasant-tasting fluoride varnishes in a simple procedure. It is therefore an ideal skill to be developed as an extended duty for dental nurses, both in the dental practice setting or on a larger scale as a public health initiative via clinics and hospital dental departments.

Patients chosen to undergo fluoride varnish application are likely to fall into one of the following categories, although oral health advice should also be given where necessary:

• Children aged 3–6 years living in areas with no water fluoridation in place
• Children aged 3–6 years showing evidence of early caries, where the caries is likely to be arrested by the fluoride application without having to have a filling placed

EXTENDED DUTIES OF THE DENTAL NURSE

- Children and young adults who are recognised as having special needs, including those requiring daily sugar-containing medications
- Children over the age of 7 years and young adults, especially those likely to develop caries due to diet, circumstance, medications, or are undergoing fixed orthodontic treatment
- Adult patients with high-risk factors for caries:
  - Active caries present at several recall appointments – this indicates an issue with poor oral hygiene or poor diet, or both
  - Dry mouth or other predisposing factors, including taking medications that cause a dry mouth as a side effect
  - Exposed roots due to gingival recession or toothbrush abrasion – root surfaces have no protective enamel covering and will develop caries more easily than the crown of the tooth
  - Extensive dental restorative work present – the margins of every restoration have the capacity to allow plaque retention to occur, increasing the risk of caries unless regular and thorough plaque removal is carried out
  - Special needs – some special needs patients may lack the manual dexterity to perform adequate plaque removal or have the inability to understand its importance, thereby having to rely on others to maintain their oral hygiene
- Adult patients with risk factors for tooth surface loss due to erosion – especially those who regularly take carbonated drinks, high-energy 'sports' drinks and some alcohols
- Adult patients with generalised dental sensitivity

Care should be taken to avoid fluorosis (overdose of fluoride systemically) with patients living in fluoridated areas (local authority or water supplier will be able to advise on this in each area) and with younger patients who are taking systemic fluoride supplements such as drops or tablets. The dentist is responsible for prescribing the application of fluoride and determining those patients who are suitable and will benefit from the procedure. The dental nurse may then apply the fluoride on their prescription.

Various fluoride varnishes are now available for the procedure (see Figure 1.4), usually as a 5% sodium fluoride varnish (this is the equivalent of 22,600 parts per million) of varying colours – obviously white varnish materials are especially popular for use rather than the dark yellow orange colour of some alternative products. Once a patient has been selected for fluoride application, and a written prescription for the procedure is recorded in their notes, the simple technique is described as follows:

TECHNIQUE:

- The dental nurse and patient wear personal protective equipment throughout the procedure
- Some patients will require specific teeth or surfaces to be treated only, while others will be prescribed a full mouth application – the notes will have been read beforehand so that the nurse follows them accurately
- Where a full mouth application is required, the mouth is treated in halves and quadrant by quadrant (so upper left, lower left, then upper right and lower right)
- Any gross plaque or tartar will have been removed previously by the dentist, therapist or hygienist – this must not be carried out on the day of fluoride application (see later)
- Most materials work best when a recent tooth polishing has been carried out beforehand, with all the prophylaxis paste removed thoroughly by the patient with copious rinsing

- Simple moisture control is achieved in each half of the mouth using either air or by wiping the relevant tooth surfaces with a cotton wool roll
- High-speed suction is not required, but the use of low-speed suction will help with tongue control when working on the lower quadrants and will make the procedure more comfortable for the patient as they do not have to keep swallowing
- The amount of fluoride varnish dispensed will depend on the number of teeth to be treated, and some products are conveniently provided in single-use dose cups of between 0.25 and 0.4g (see Figure 1.4) – no more than one dose cup should be used per application, and any remaining product must be disposed of rather than used on another patient
- The dispensed fluoride varnish is stirred to ensure an even consistency throughout, and then carefully applied to the required tooth surfaces using a micro-brush (Figure 14.8)
- The varnish should not come into contact with the gums during application
- Where a preventive, full-mouth application is undertaken the varnish is applied to all pits, fissures and each contact point in each quadrant
- Once the full quadrant has been treated, the varnish is allowed to become moist either naturally with saliva or by gentle rinsing – this thickens the varnish to a more gel-like consistency and enables the material to remain in place for several hours
- The procedure is repeated in all required areas according to the individual prescription from the dentist
- The patient is given the following verbal post-operative instructions, and a written handout reiterating the points, to take home
- Avoid eating, drinking or toothbrushing for a minimum of 30 minutes
- Have a soft-food diet for the remainder of the day
- Avoid the use of mouthwashes for the remainder of the day, particularly those containing fluoride or alcohol
- The varnish will slough off naturally over the next few days – this is not an issue as the preventive action begins immediately upon contact with the tooth
- The application process can be repeated every 3–6 months as required

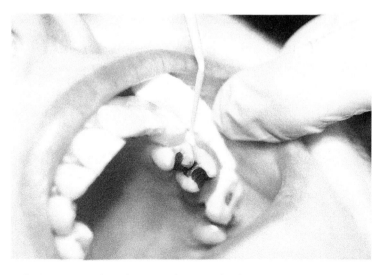

Figure 14.8 Fluoride varnish application with a micro-brush, avoiding contact with the gum tissue

PRECAUTIONS AND CONTRAINDICATIONS

Fluoride varnish is intended for use as a topical application, directly to the outer surface of the tooth or root and not as a systemic application, taken internally. It should therefore not be used on children under 3 years of age who are most likely to swallow some of the product during application. Fluoride overdose (fluorosis) is also a potential hazard in patients taking other fluoride supplements at the time of application, and they must be advised accordingly.

Fluoride application is contraindicated (not advisable) in all patients with ulcerative gingivitis or stomatitis and should not be used when any level of gingival inflammation is present (such as immediately after gross scaling) as the fluoride can gain systemic entry to the blood stream and the body through these inflamed tissues. One of its constituents may also cause hypersensitivity or even allergic reaction in susceptible patients and is therefore not to be used in patients diagnosed with bronchial asthma, or other allergy-like reactions requiring hospital admission. Finally, as with many other medicaments, the effects of fluoride on the foetus or newborn are unknown and consequently, fluoride application in pregnant or nursing mothers is strongly inadvisable.

For the vast majority of patients then, regular and targeted fluoride varnish application is an extremely useful technique in the prevention or control of early caries and dental hypersensitivity. A suitably trained dental nurse carrying out the procedure under prescription is an asset to the dental team, able to assist many patients of all ages to prevent future problems while allowing other team members to proceed with more advanced oral health care procedures.

FURTHER SKILLS IN ASSISTING IN THE TREATMENT OF ORTHODONTIC PATIENTS

Most orthodontic treatment is carried out in specialist practices or clinics in the United Kingdom, so many dental nurses have little or no access to the speciality in general practice. Of those dental nurses who do work within the orthodontic speciality, one with extended duties in this area of dentistry is a valuable member of the team in delivering this treatment, along with the dentist and the orthodontic therapist. The extended duties that can be developed include any and all of the following:

- Recognition and laying out of the specialised orthodontic instruments and materials – although this area of dentistry is included in the dental nurse curriculum of the registerable qualification, the knowledge required is only to a basic level
- Setting up of brackets and tubes for the bonding of fixed appliances
- Specific oral hygiene instruction for orthodontic patients
- Measurement and recording of plaque indices before, during and after treatment (this skill can be gained as a separate extended duty; see later)
- Tracing cephalographs (this skill can be gained as a separate extended duty; see later)

Laying out instruments and materials

The majority of orthodontic treatments carried out on younger patients in the United Kingdom (via the NHS) involve the use of removable, functional or conventional fixed appliances (see Chapter 12 for further details). Many of the instruments and materials

EXTENDED DUTIES OF THE DENTAL NURSE

required for the fitting/bonding, adjustment and removal of these appliances are unique to this speciality and are therefore unlikely to be familiar to many dental nurses. The following table lists the most likely instruments to be required for removable and functional appliances (see Figure 12.2) and conventional fixed appliances (see Figure 12.4) and their functions. Those to be laid out will be determined by the appliance involved and the stage of the treatment that is being undertaken.

Item	Function
Adam pliers	Removable/functional appliance – to tighten cribs, adjust springs and retractors
Straight hand piece with acrylic bur	Removable/functional appliance – to trim the acrylic base plate of the appliance
Measuring ruler	All appliances – to take accurate measurements of tooth movements, such as the overjet
Bracket holders (see Figure 12.6b)	Fixed appliance – to pick up, hold and position individual brackets during their bonding onto the teeth
Alastik/elastic holders (see Figure 12.6c)	Fixed appliance – ratcheted design to pick up and tightly grip alastiks and elastics as they are used to tie in the arch wire to the bracket (alastik) or to provide traction to teeth (elastics)
Arch wire (end) cutters (see Figure 12.6d)	Fixed appliance – angled wire cutters to trim off the excess ends of the arch wire from directly behind the molar band or tube, often with a self-gripping attachment so that the cut piece of wire can be safely removed from the mouth
Wire cutters (Figure 14.9a)	Fixed appliance – straight wire cutters to trim off the ends of wire ties or ligatures
Bracket removers (Figure 14.9b)	Fixed appliance – chisel-ended pliers to remove brackets from the teeth at the end of treatment or when a bracket requires removing and repositioning
Band removers (Figure 14.9c)	Fixed appliance – chisel-ended blade and a plastic stopper to remove bands at the end of treatment; the stopper rests on the occlusal surface of the tooth while the other blade is located at the gingival rim of the band, and then the pliers are squeezed together to dislodge the band from the tooth

The materials that may be required to be laid out are as follows:

- Alginate impression material and water for pre- and post-operative study models, and for the working model when a removable appliance is to be constructed (see Figure 4.22)
- Acid etch and a suitable bonding agent when a fixed appliance is to be placed (see Figure 12.6a)
- Suitable luting cement for the cementation of molar bands

Setting up for a bonding procedure

Bonding a conventional fixed appliance to an upper, lower or both arches is a fiddly and sometimes time-consuming procedure, and forward preparation is a key element in the smooth running of the appointment, for both the patient and the dentist.

EXTENDED DUTIES OF THE DENTAL NURSE

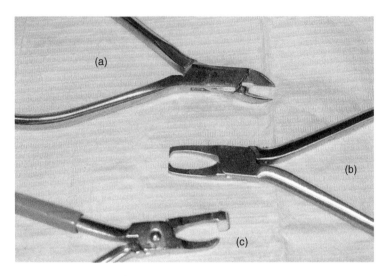

Figure 14.9 Fixed appliance instruments. (a) Wire cutters. (b) Bracket removers. (c) Band removers

    The dental nurse can assist greatly by being trained to set out the brackets and molar tubes beforehand. This is best done using an orientation card with a sticky backing on which the brackets and tubes can be firmly located, ready for the procedure. Each bracket and tube are designed for use on a specific tooth only and great care must be taken in orientating each one correctly. Brackets have coloured dots placed on their disto-gingival wing by the manufacturers to assist in their identification, but the colours used may vary between suppliers, so bracket sets should not become mixed together. The exception is lower incisor brackets that have a rounded base that follows the gingival margin of the tooth but can otherwise be used on any of the lower incisors. Canine brackets can also have disto-gingival hooks placed by the manufacturer for use with elastic traction. Molar tubes have distally orientated hooks that are set gingivally, so upper right molar tubes can also be used on lower left molars, and upper left molar tubes can also be used on lower right molars.

    When placing the brackets, the dental nurse should use the bracket holders so that they become familiar with their use and handling.

    Examples of the various features of the brackets and tubes discussed are shown in Figure 14.10.

Orthodontic oral hygiene instruction

Both removable and fixed appliances provide many more stagnation areas in the patient's mouth than would exist without the appliance in situ, and the high level of oral hygiene that must be maintained throughout the treatment is imperative if tooth damage and localised gingival problems are to be avoided. The patient must be taught how and when to clean adequately around the appliance, as well as any necessary dietary controls to be followed during the treatment phase – this oral hygiene instruction can be delivered by a suitably trained dental nurse. In addition, patients who have fixed appliances placed are deemed to be at high risk for developing caries and should therefore undergo fluoride

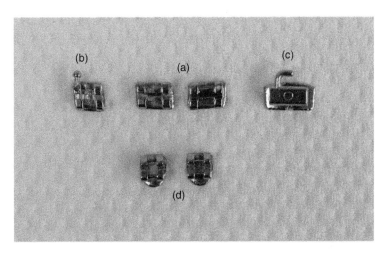

Figure 14.10 Examples of fixed appliance components. (a) Upper right and left brackets with orientation dots. (b) Upper right canine bracket with hook. (c) Upper left molar tube. (d) Lower incisor bracket with rounded base

application every 3 months during the treatment course – this is another extended duty that can be carried out by a suitably trained dental nurse (see previously).

Over and above any general oral hygiene advice and instruction which is relevant to all patients, that advice and instruction specific to those wearing removable appliances is as follows:

- Food and drink must be confined to mealtimes rather than having snacks throughout the day, as the teeth will need cleaning every time something has been consumed so that food debris is not held against the teeth by the appliance
- The quantity of food and drink containing free sugars and acids must be kept to an absolute minimum to reduce the potential of causing cavities during treatment
- The appliance must be removed and cleaned twice daily with a toothbrush and toothpaste, taking care not to damage any springs or clasps while doing so
- Cleaning should be carried out over a sink of water so that if dropped, the appliance will not break
- Both fluoride mouthwash and toothpaste should be used during the treatment phase on a daily basis, to provide maximum protection against caries to the teeth
- Patients should be encouraged to self-disclose their teeth on a weekly basis to ensure their oral hygiene regime is adequate
- If extraction spaces are present in the dental arch, the patient should be instructed in the use of an interspace brush to clean the area effectively until space closure occurs

Over and above any general oral hygiene advice and instruction which is relevant to all patients, that advice and instruction specific to those wearing fixed appliances is as follows:

- The quantity of food and drink containing free sugars and acids must be kept to an absolute minimum to reduce the potential of causing cavities during treatment

- Both fluoride mouthwash and toothpaste should be used during the treatment phase on a daily basis to provide maximum protection against caries to the teeth
- Ideally, patients should be encouraged to check the effectiveness of their oral hygiene efforts by using disclosing tablets regularly but, as the elastic components of the fixed appliance will be permanently discoloured by them, their use is best confined to just before a scheduled appointment with the dentist so that the discoloured elastics can be changed
- Patients should be instructed in the use of interdental brushes to clean around each bracket where the arch wire passes over, as this is a particular stagnation area where ordinary manual tooth brushing alone is not sufficient (see Figure 12.11)
- Alternatively, the patient can be instructed in the use of an electric toothbrush with an orthodontic head attachment to clean these areas

In either form of orthodontic treatment, if a less than adequate level of oral hygiene is being maintained by the patient, the dental nurse can provide a one-to-one disclosing and cleaning session to emphasise the problem areas and help the patient to improve their plaque removal.

Measurement and recording of plaque indices

A plaque index is a method used to measure the amount of plaque present in the patient's mouth at any time – the higher the index, the greater the amount of plaque present. When carried out repeatedly over several visits, it provides a record of a patient's progress in their oral hygiene standards. So, it allows a numerical value to be placed on the level of oral hygiene at that point, which can then be used to monitor progress over a period of time – and the use of a numerical value makes the information more understandable to the patients; they can quantify their own progress. Plaque indices can be used for any patient but are particularly useful with potential and ongoing orthodontic patients because they provide information that can be used in the following ways:

- A high plaque index in a potential orthodontic patient prevents the start of treatment until improvement is seen – it therefore 'weeds out' unsuitable patients who are most likely to develop caries if treatment would have proceeded otherwise
- It gives the patient something to aim for if they desire orthodontic treatment – to reduce the numerical value to an acceptable level
- It monitors the compliance of the patient during treatment – if problems are identified, they can be resolved before tooth damage occurs
- If problems continue, the treatment can be abandoned with a recorded (and therefore irrefutable) good reason, and hopefully before tooth damage occurs
- When treatment has been successfully completed, a lowered index provides a retrospective record of the need for the treatment initially – the patient's oral hygiene has improved as cleaning became easier as their teeth became well-aligned during the orthodontic treatment

Two established methods are available for measuring and recording the amount of plaque present in the patient's mouth – one method involves every tooth present, while the other involves just six teeth as a representative sample of the mouth as a whole and is therefore a speedier procedure.

METHOD 1

- Assume each tooth is divided into six sites – mesial, mid and distal on both the buccal and lingual/palatal sides
- Multiply the number of teeth present in the patient's mouth by six – a typical teenager is likely to have all but their third molars present, so 28 teeth × 6 = 168
- The presence or absence of plaque at each site is determined by running a blunt probe along the gingival margins of each tooth, or by thoroughly disclosing the patient and looking directly at the teeth
- Total the number of sites (out of 168) where plaque is present – so say 102 sites out of 168 had plaque present, 102/168
- Multiply this fraction by 100 to give a percentage plaque index = 60.7%

A high plaque index indicates the patient has a poor standard of oral hygiene and is not suitable for orthodontic treatment until the plaque index has been much reduced and then maintained at a reduced level consistently. So, the quantified information can be used to motivate a keen patient to improve their oral hygiene, or to justify the denial of treatment to an insistent patient who has little interest in improving their oral hygiene but wants orthodontic treatment anyway.

METHOD 2

- Six teeth are chosen as a representative sample of the mouth – the upper right first molar (UR6, 16) and lateral incisor (UR2, 12), and the upper left first premolar (UL4, 24); the lower left first molar (LL6, 36) and lateral incisor (LL2, 32), and the lower right first premolar (LR4, 44)
- The presence or absence of plaque is determined on four sites of each tooth – mesial and distal of both the buccal and lingual/palatal sides
- The plaque is scored as follows:
  - No plaque = 0
  - Plaque present by probing = 1
  - Visible plaque = 2
  - Extensive plaque = 3
- The average plaque scores of each tooth are added together and then divided by six (the number of teeth that have been recorded) to give a single figure which is taken as a representative average for the mouth as a whole – this is the patient's plaque index
- So using the following example:
  - UR6 = 2
  - UR2 = 0
  - UL4 = 2
  - LL6 = 3
  - LL2 = 3
  - LR4 = 2
- Total = 12 ÷ 6 = plaque index 2
- Using this qualitative and quicker method, the plaque index will range from 0 (excellent) to 3 (poor), so again this patient is currently unsuitable for orthodontic treatment

The plaque index can be calculated by the dental nurse at any point during treatment and compared with the pre-operative scores to monitor the oral hygiene progress of the patient and highlight any potential problems as they occur and before any tooth damage is likely to have happened. The plaque index can be recorded at the examination or recall appointment of any patient, not just those considering orthodontic treatment, and is a useful method of monitoring routine oral hygiene standards and the patient's compliance with any previous oral hygiene instruction given.

Methods of recording the information to determine the plaque index vary widely, but probably one of the simplest ways is to use a preprinted dental arch diagram with dots to indicate the presence of plaque (method 1; Figure 14.11a). Alternatively, a variation of a standard periodontal diagnosis and treatment plan chart can be used. The chart has the buccal, lingual, and palatal surfaces of each tooth pre-printed onto it, and plaque can be recorded as either a dot at each site (method 1) or as a numerical value at each site and then take the average for the tooth (method 2; Figure 14.11b).

A post-registration qualification in Orthodontic Dental Nursing is available for dental nurses in the United Kingdom, which trains students to a much greater depth in this speciality and is particularly useful for those dental nurses wishing to work in a specialist orthodontic workplace. Further details are available at www.nebdn.org.

TRACING CEPHALOGRAPHS

In simple terms, a cephalograph is a tracing made from a lateral skull radiograph which is used in orthodontics for various reasons:

- To help determine the skeletal pattern of the patient before orthodontic treatment begins
- To help determine the likelihood for orthognathic surgery to correct more severe orthodontic cases
- To monitor the skull and jaw growth of the patient
- To assess skeletal changes that have occurred due to orthodontic treatment and natural growth

While the skill of tracing the various points on the cephalograph is a useful extended duty to hold by dental nurses working in specialist orthodontic environments, the interpretation of the findings is for the dentist to understand and act upon. Consequently, only the basics of tracing skills are discussed here.

The typical lateral skull radiograph image (see Figure 4.15) is produced as a two-dimensional 'side view' of the patient's skull, with no horizontal distortion – so the ear-pieces used to hold the patient's head still during X-ray exposure are superimposed directly over each other and appear as one on the image.

Once the radiograph has been processed (or printed off as a hard copy if a digital technique is used) the image is taped to an X-ray viewing screen and overlaid with either a taped sheet of tracing paper or a taped sheet of acetate film, which is more durable. Taping the radiograph and overlay in place prevents unwanted movements during tracing and therefore produces a more accurate result.

Using a hard pencil or a fine felt-tip pen, the soft tissue outline of the patient's face is traced from the radiograph followed by the following features, all shown in red in Figure 14.12:

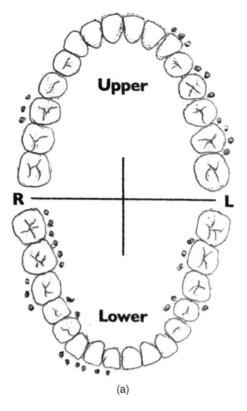

(a)

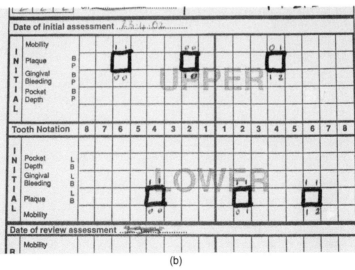

(b)

Figure 14.11 Examples of plaque index recording methods. (a) Preprinted dental arches with dots (method 1). (b) Variation of standard periodontal chart with numerical scores (method 2)

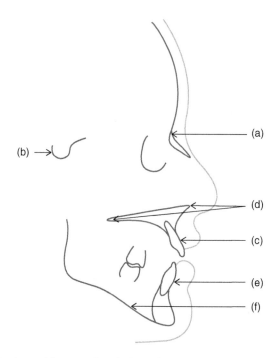

Figure 14.12 Initial traced features of cephalograph

- The junction of the frontal bone with the nasal bone (a)
- Sella turcica: the bony depression in the sphenoid bone where the pituitary gland lies (b)
- Outline of the upper central incisor in the alveolar ridge (c)
- Anterior and posterior nasal spines of the palate (d)
- Outline of the lower central incisor in the alveolar ridge (e)
- Lower border of the mandible to the ramus (f)

With these features traced, the following points can then be marked on the cephalograph (the anatomical descriptions have been simplified where possible), all shown in blue in Figure 14.13:

- Point S – the centre-point of the sella turcica
- Point N – the nasion, the most anterior point of the frontonasal suture (at the bridge of the nose)
- Point A – the deepest point of the upper alveolar ridge
- Point B – the deepest point of the lower alveolar ridge

Finally, the maxillary plane can be drawn in as a line between the anterior and posterior nasal spines, and the mandibular plane can be drawn in as a line representing the lower border of the mandible; both are shown in green in Figure 14.13.

EXTENDED DUTIES OF THE DENTAL NURSE

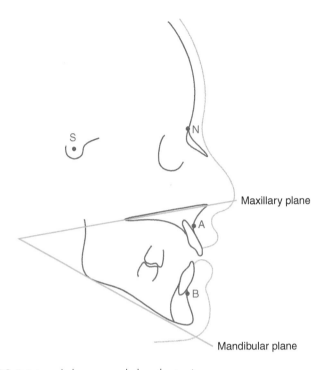

Figure 14.13 Points and planes recorded on the tracing

The radiograph is removed from the viewer so that just the tracing remains, lines are then drawn between the various anatomical points, and the necessary angles are measured to provide the cephalography information for orthodontic analysis:

- SNA angle
- SNB angle
- ANB angle
- M/M angle (maxillary/mandibular planes angle)

A completed tracing with the angles measured is shown in Figure 14.14. This can then be passed to the dentist for analysis.

TAKING IMPRESSIONS

Alginate impressions are the most frequently taken and widely useful of the impression materials available. They are used to produce study models in various fields of dentistry, to produce opposing models and initial models in fixed and removable prosthodontics, and to produce models for the construction of mouth guards, vacuum-formed retainers and whitening trays (see later).

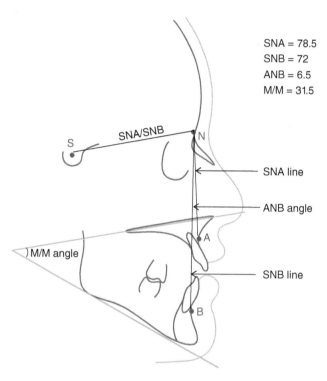

SNA = 78.5
SNB = 72
ANB = 6.5
M/M = 31.5

Figure 14.14 Completed tracing of cephalograph

A trained and competent dental nurse who can take consistently good quality and therefore useful alginate impressions is an asset to any dental workplace. The stages involved in taking alginate impressions are as follows:

- Selection of the patient – many patients are fearful of undergoing impression taking, as they believe they will choke, gag, or vomit, and excessively fearful patients are best left to the dentist to handle
- Selection of the trays
- Mixing of the alginate and loading of the trays
- Insertion of the loaded trays
- Removal of the trays after setting
- Monitoring and handling of the patient throughout

The equipment and materials required to take a set of study models are shown in Figure 4.22.

Selection of the trays

It is usual for single-use, perforated box trays to be used for alginate impression taking, with the correct tray handle inserted before use if the tray design is one without a handle already incorporated. Tray handles should always be used as they provide the operator with good leverage during tray removal, otherwise the trays may be difficult to remove once the alginate has set with time.

Suitably sized trays should just fit over the dental arch in either jaw, without being excessively wide (they will be difficult to insert through the oral aperture of the lips), without being excessively long (they need to go no further posteriorly than the end of the dental arch), and without being excessively short (they must record the full length of the dental arch). A trial tray insertion must always be carried out on the patient before proceeding with the impression taking to avoid poor quality impressions, which will need to be retaken. When a chosen tray has been inserted, it should be lifted up and down over the dental arch – if there is any catching on the teeth, or any resistance to being fully seated, then the tray is too narrow (Figure 14.15a and b).

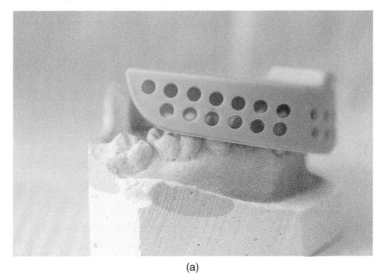

(a)

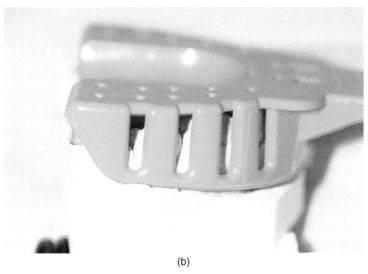

(b)

Figure 14.15 Sizing of tray for impression taking. (a) Tray is catching molar teeth: too narrow. (b) Correct tray size: just covering the dental arch

Usually, upper trays are used for upper impressions and lowers for lower impressions. However, on occasions when the palate does not need to be recorded (such as with retainers and bleaching trays), a suitably sized lower tray may be used in the upper arch, and this is also less likely to stimulate a gag reflex in some patients.

Mixing of the alginate and loading of the trays

All dental nurses are familiar with the correct mixing of alginate, and the technique is summarised as follows:

- Ensure the powder measuring scoop and the water measure are for the same material, otherwise the 1:1 powder to water proportions will be incorrect, resulting in either too stiff a mix or a sloppy mix
- Shake the powder container to mix the contents, ensuring the container lid is firmly closed beforehand
- Use full and levelled scoops of powder, usually two are required for each impression
- Make a well in the powder in the mixing bowl and pour the measured room temperature water into the centre of the well (Figure 14.16a)
- Fold the powder into the water initially then vigorously mix and spatulate the mixture against the sides of the bowl (Figure 14.16b)
- Ensure all the powder is mixed in and that no air bubbles have been introduced into the mix – when fully mixed the alginate should have a uniform consistency (Figure 14.16c)

Upper trays are loaded with the full mix gathered on the spatula, and from the back of the tray forwards so that it is loaded uniformly across its whole width and length (Figure 14.16d).

Lower trays are loaded in two stages, with half the mix gathered on the spatula for each. The first half of the mix is loaded into one half of the tray from the inner side of the tray arch, and the second half into the other side (Figure 14.16e) so that the tray is equally filled with the impression material.

Insertion of the trays

Each impression is mixed, loaded, inserted and removed one at a time. The insertion technique is as follows:

- The patient wears a waterproof bib and sits upright in the dental chair
- The patient is instructed to relax the lips and to breathe at a normal rate through the nose while the impression is in the mouth
- The lower impression is inserted while standing in front of the patient, by angling the loaded tray so one end passes through the oral aperture first and then is swung over to that side of the dental arch before seating – this brings the other side of the tray through the oral aperture and over the other side of the dental arch
- A right-handed dental nurse will find the process easier if the left side of the tray is inserted first, and the left hand is used to gently retract the lips as the right side is inserted later (and the opposite for a left-handed dental nurse)
- Once the full tray is hovering over the full lower arch, it is gently pushed down onto the teeth, ensuring that the teeth are in the centre of the tray all around the arch (so not too close to either the buccal or lingual side of the tray)

- The lower lip may be pulled out and 'rolled' up over the front of the tray to ensure the labial sulcus is fully recorded
- The patient is asked to raise their tongue once the impression is seated, then to move it from one side to the other, then finally to stick their tongue out to touch their top teeth or lip – these movements ensure the lingual margins of the impression are recorded accurately
- The tray is held evenly in this position with the fingers by the dental nurse until setting occurs, in particular, it must be held firm if the patient swallows as the tray would lift up otherwise

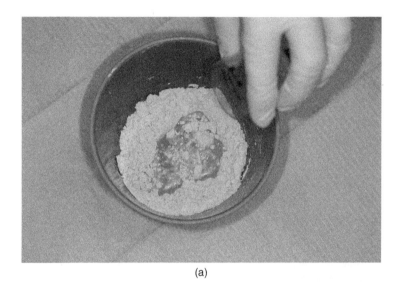

(a)

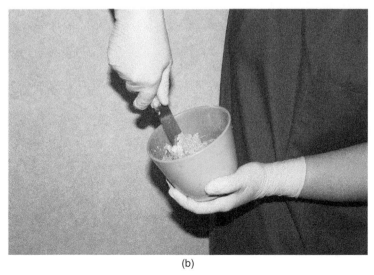

(b)

Figure 14.16 (a–e) Alginate mixing and tray loading

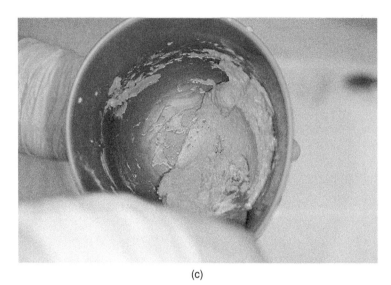

(c)

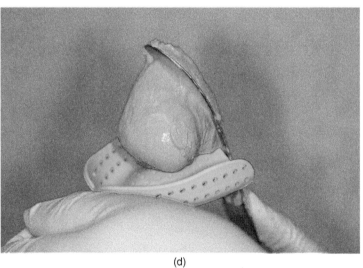

(d)

Figure 14.16 (*continued*)

- The upper impression is inserted while standing behind the patient, to the right (for a right-handed dental nurse), or to the left (for a left-handed dental nurse)
- Again, the tray is inserted by angling first one side, and then the other through the oral aperture while retracting the lips with the other hand (right side first for a right-handed dental nurse)
- Once the full tray is hovering below the full upper arch, it is gently pushed up onto the teeth, from the back forwards to prevent material from being pushed into the patient's throat

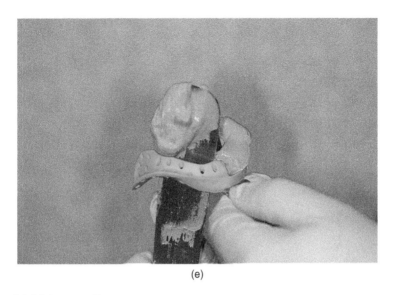

(e)

Figure 14.16 (continued)

- Again, ensure that the teeth are in the centre of the tray all around the arch
- The upper lip may be pulled out and 'rolled' down over the front of the tray to ensure the labial sulcus is fully recorded
- The tray is supported evenly in this position with the fingers until setting occurs

Removal of the trays after setting

Any excess impression material can be squeezed to determine if the setting has occurred – that in the patient's mouth will have set quicker still because the oral cavity is a warmer environment. Otherwise, the impression material lying in either labial sulcus can be touched to determine if it has fully set – it should feel firm and not leave any impression material on the gloves when the finger is pulled away.

Once set, the trays are removed after loosening the cheeks by running a finger around the buccal and labial sulci, then exerting a firm upward pressure on the tray handle of the lower tray, and a firm downward pressure on the tray handle of the upper tray. The impression can then be gradually eased over the teeth and out of the mouth, reversing the angle and swing action of the insertion process so that the patient's soft tissues are not uncomfortably stretched.

On removal, the impression should be checked for accuracy before being sent for disinfection – if it is not adequate, then the impression taking must be repeated. For example, the impression shown in Figure 14.17 has well-rolled edges and no air blows, but the upper right molar tooth has not been fully recorded in the impression, and this may require a retake.

If the impressions are acceptable, they are disinfected in the usual manner – rinsed, soaked, rinsed, packaged with damp gauze in a sealed bag, and correctly labelled with the patient and job details, plus a label confirming the disinfection date.

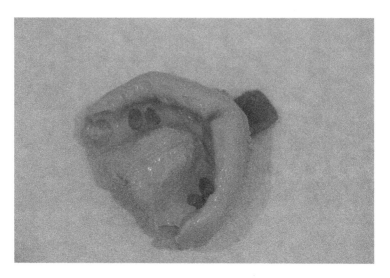

Figure 14.17 Example of an upper alginate impression

Monitoring and handling of the patient

Suitable personal protective equipment must be provided and worn by the patient, and the dental nurse must wear clinical gloves throughout the whole procedure. The dental nurse must always be aware of the fear and trepidation that some patients may exhibit when told they require impressions to be taken, and they should be empathetic to the patient's concerns. Any overly anxious patient should be referred to the dentist.

Some patients prefer to know what is involved in the procedure beforehand, others prefer not. Where possible a short and simplified explanation should be given to all patients; in particular, the following points should be mentioned:

- The material sets relatively quickly, and the impressions will be removed as soon as possible
- Stay calm and breathe at a normal rate through the nose throughout the procedure
- If they begin to panic and try to remove the trays, their mouth will be covered in unset impression material which is difficult to remove – they must concentrate on their breathing and allow the procedure to continue
- Allow the lips to remain relaxed so that they can be retracted and manipulated as necessary by the dental nurse
- Follow the tongue instructions carefully
- Once the impressions are in place, they may tip their heads forward if they wish – this reduces the choking fear
- Do not worry if they begin dribbling while the impression is still inserted and setting – the waterproof bib will prevent any clothing damage
- Some considerable effort may be required to remove the impressions in some patients (because they have undercuts that 'lock' the impression in place), but it is *not* enough to pull their teeth out
- Give a distraction technique if necessary to overly anxious patients – for example, ask them to concentrate and count backward from three hundred in 3's in their mind once the trays are in place (so 300, 297, 294, 291, and so on)

EXTENDED DUTIES OF THE DENTAL NURSE

During the procedure, the dental nurse should also remain calm and in control of the situation. Make encouraging comments throughout ('you're doing really well', 'we've nearly finished now', 'well done', and so on).

Once the impressions are removed, the dental nurse should help the patient to have a rinse and then check and remove any extra-oral impression material from the patient's facial area – never send the patient away looking like a mess. Also, check if any impression tags are stuck between their teeth and provide floss for the patient to dislodge it. Congratulate them on 'surviving' the ordeal and reiterate how well they did.

POURING, CASTING AND TRIMMING STUDY MODELS

Study models enable the dentist to study the patient's dentition and occlusion outside the mouth and from all angles – this 'extra dimension' is often invaluable in determining diagnoses, and issues that were not obvious simply by looking in the mouth. They are particularly useful for orthodontic assessments, occlusal analyses, partial denture design, and as a permanent record of the dentition at a point in time when conditions such as non-carious tooth surface loss are being monitored. They are produced as stone casts poured into alginate impressions and are usually made in the dental laboratory. However, where many study model sets are required in the dental workplace on a regular basis, the task can be carried out by the dental nurse on the premises following adequate training, so that the models are produced more speedily and at a much-reduced cost to the workplace. In addition, accurate study models can be produced as soon as the alginate impressions have been taken and disinfected on the premises, rather than awaiting collection and transfer to the laboratory some days later.

There are three stages to the production of a set of study models:

- *Pouring* – the initial accurate filling of each disinfected alginate impression with a flowable mix of dental stone material to record the tooth and soft tissue detail of each arch
- *Casting* – the shaping of the study model itself by the hardening (setting) of the dental stone within the mould of the alginate impression
- *Trimming* – the addition and accurate trimming of plaster bases to the study models in their correct occlusion, so that the study model set can stand alone and be viewed from all angles with the teeth recorded in their actual bite positions

Pouring

The alginate impressions and bite record (either a simple wax bite record or a full arch bite registration – see Figure 14.18) are disinfected in the usual manner, and then any excess fluid is removed from their surface by careful shaking of the impressions into the sink. Excess fluid droplets on the alginate surface are likely to result in air blows and a poor dental stone surface on the model if not removed.

Dental stone is a hardened, calcium-based plaster material that does not react with impression materials and is able to reproduce fine detail and sharp margins when set – so the study models produced are very accurate. Coloured dies are usually added to the material; yellow for study models and pink, blue or green for even harder products used for crown and bridge work.

EXTENDED DUTIES OF THE DENTAL NURSE

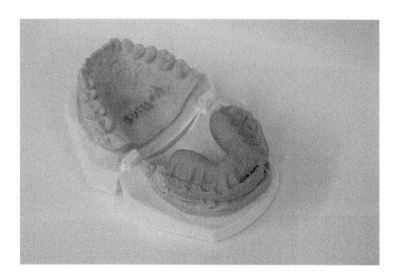

Figure 14.18 Bite record using a putty and catalyst material

Although a conventional alginate mixing bowl and spatula can be used to mix the stone, the technique is quite different from that used to mix alginate (see previously). The mixed dental stone must have the following properties to provide an accurate casting of the impression:

- Correct water: powder ratio to produce a flowable mix that can be poured into the impression
- No lumps of unmixed powder present
- No excess water present
- No air bubbles present

Unfortunately, achieving the correct mixing ratio comes with experience rather than by measuring a set weight of powder and mixing it with a set volume of water – differences in manufacturer alone create variable mixes. Fortunately, dental stone is inexpensive, and practice makes perfect!

Dental stone is mixed and poured as follows:

- Cold water is run into the mixing bowl – the volume depends on whether the two study models are being cast from one mix or two mixes, but as an average use 50 ml
- The powder is sifted onto the top of the water and allowed to sink in until only a little free water remains (Figure 14.19)
- The powder and water are then carefully **folded** together to create a smooth slurry consistency, with no lumps of powder or unmixed water remaining (Figure 14.20)
- Stirring and spatulation actions such as those used to mix alginate must **not** be used to mix the stone, as this will incorporate air bubbles into the mix
- A vibration plate can be used to ensure that air bubbles are removed from the mix before pouring, but holding the mixing bowl lightly on the top of the ultrasonic bath while running provides an adequate alternative method

EXTENDED DUTIES OF THE DENTAL NURSE

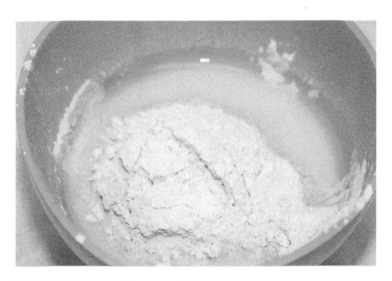

Figure 14.19 Sifted stone powder in water before mixing

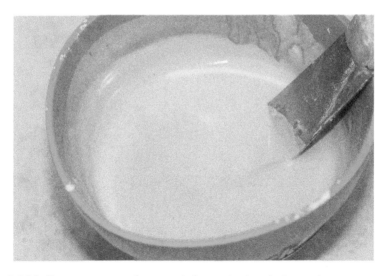

Figure 14.20 Slurry consistency of mix, ready for pouring into the impression

- When ready, the flowable mix is poured into the impression at either the right or left most distal tooth, and then the tray is tipped to allow the mix to flow from this point around the full arch to the other distal tooth in one motion – this tends to push air before it and out of the impression recesses as the mix flows around the impression (Figure 14.21)
- The mix should fill the impression to above the gingival margins of the teeth and be prevented from pouring out of the back of the impression by raising its level and supporting the back of the tray if necessary (Figure 14.22)

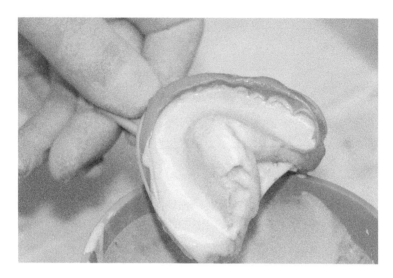

Figure 14.21 Running the stone mix around the impression to eliminate air trapping

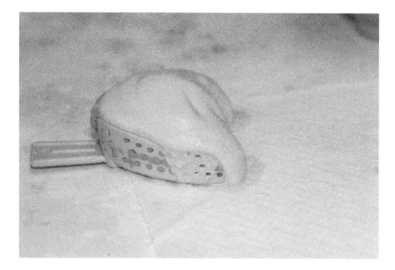

Figure 14.22 Filled impression kept level during setting to avoid run-off

Casting

At this point, more powder can be added to any unused mix to make a stiffer dental stone, which can be carefully loaded onto the top of the impression – this produces a more robust model for handling later, rather than a weak horse-shoe shaped rim recording the teeth only, which is likely to fracture when removed from the impression. The 'construction' produced can either be left in this position to set fully, or it can be turned upside down so that the stiffer mix forms a flat base to the cast (Figure 14.23). Either way, care must be taken to ensure that the mix does not come into contact with the edges

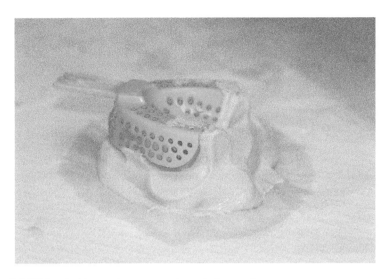

Figure 14.23 Loaded impression on stone base during casting

of the impression tray itself during setting, as this will make it difficult to remove the tray and impression later without fracturing the teeth of the casting produced.

The setting reaction is exothermic (gives off heat), and the dental stone will feel warm to the touch. Once the casting is cold to the touch it can be assumed that setting is complete, but it is best to leave the casting untouched for several hours to ensure full setting has occurred.

The easiest way of ensuring that the casting does not fracture as it is removed from the impression is to remove the tray first, using an instrument such as a spatula or wax knife to lever it off the casting while leaving the impression intact (Figure 14.24). The revealed

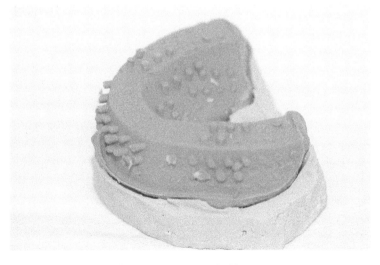

Figure 14.24 Tray removed before impression is peeled from casting

impression can then be carefully peeled off the model in pieces so that tooth fractures are avoided. Although this destroys the impression, if the casting produced is faulty (such as having air blows present), the impression could not have been re-used anyway, and a new impression will be required.

Trimming

The dental stone castings now need to be positioned together in their correct occlusion so that they can be viewed by the dentist in a reproducible position while diagnoses and treatment plans are formulated. This involves placing the bite registration so that the castings occlude correctly, then seating them into pre-shaped plastic bases loaded with dental plaster which, once set, allows the study models to be viewed separately and then repositioned into their correct occlusion time and time again. Alternatively, the castings are seated onto un-shaped mounds of plaster and then shaped manually using a trimming machine. In either technique, the base of the lower model must be parallel to the occlusal plane so that the models are not set in a 'tipped' position. Dental plaster is used as it is not as hard as dental stone and therefore easier to trim using a carborundum wheel trimming machine – this technique was often used in the dental laboratory, while that using pre-shaped plastic bases with alignment tags (Figure 14.25) tends to be used now both in the laboratory and the dental workplace. The key to success is to ensure that the back edges of the pre-shaped bases are exactly in line with each other during setting and with the bite registration in place using the alignment tags, so that the study models can only be placed in their correct positions once the bases are set.

Dental plaster is mixed in the same way as dental stone but to a much stiffer consistency which can support the casting while the plaster base sets, without the casting sinking into it.

Once the final set of study models has been trimmed accordingly, they can be used by the dentist as necessary (see Figure 4.21).

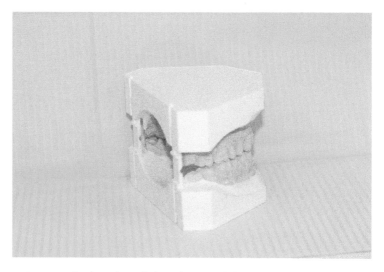

Figure 14.25 Example of pre-shaped plastic bases and alignment tags used to complete the study model set

CONSTRUCTING BLEACHING TRAYS

Bleaching trays, mouth guards, and vacuum-formed retainers are constructed in a similar process to each other, the difference being the material used for each one. The technique used to construct bleaching trays is described. These are devices made for patients to use at home when carrying out tooth whitening (see Chapter 13). Mouth guards are worn by patients who have a bruxing habit (tooth clenching and grinding habit) that is causing tooth wear and/or tooth fracture, or jaw joint discomfort, and vacuum-formed retainers are the gum shield-type retainers worn by patients after completing a course of orthodontic treatment (see Chapter 12).

Each device is made by pulling a warmed sheet of varying thickness rubbery material, called EVA tray material, over a stone model of the patient's dental arch, which is then sucked tightly onto the model under vacuum. Bleaching trays are made from very thin EVA sheets, while orthodontic retainers and mouth guards are constructed from thicker materials.

Once the tray has been removed from the model and carefully trimmed, a unique device is produced that is a perfect fit over the patient's own teeth. As the fit is so accurate, it cannot be placed into the mouth in any but the correct position (so it is easy for the patient to wear), it fits tightly but comfortably onto the teeth (so it does not fall out or become loose), and the material used is transparent so the device is not obvious.

An example of a vacuum machine used for the tray construction is shown in Figure 14.26.

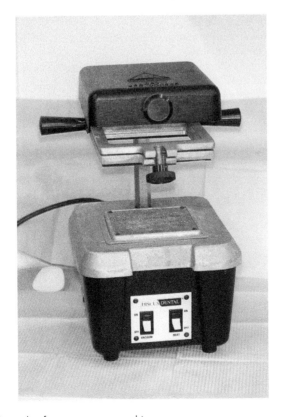

Figure 14.26 Example of a vacuum tray machine

The technique for producing the bleaching tray is as follows:

- The stone models of the dental arches to be bleached are provided by the laboratory, or cast up on-site by the dental nurse as an extended duty
- They are trimmed to remove the sulci areas, and upper models have the palate removed or a hole placed through so that the suction under vacuum can be applied to all sides of the model equally during the tray-forming process
- The teeth to be bleached (this varies between patients) have a spacer material present on the labial surfaces, so that a well is formed during tray construction for the application of the bleaching gel – the spacer in the images used is hard blue wax
- The model is placed on the base of the machine and a sheet of EVA loaded and locked into the tray reservoir above it (Figure 14.27)
- The heater above the tray material is switched on to warm the sheet – it is ready to be pulled over the model when the warmed sheet hangs about 1.5 cm below the reservoir (Figure 14.28)
- The tray reservoir is pulled sharply down to the bottom of the machine so that it lies over the model, and the vacuum is switched on immediately (the heater can be switched off at this point)
- The suction produced pulls the sheet tightly over the model to produce the tray – the vacuum should be left to run for a minimum of 30 seconds
- Once the construction is complete, the machine is switched off and the model and tray are left to cool before handling
- Bleaching trays are carefully trimmed to follow the gingival line of the teeth, producing a scalloped edge (see Figure 13.2)
- Orthodontic retainers and mouth guards are trimmed to leave a 2 mm extension beyond the gingival margins, so that the tray edge lies on the gingivae
- The trimmed edges are smoothed to avoid any soft tissue trauma – an emery board or similar file is ideal

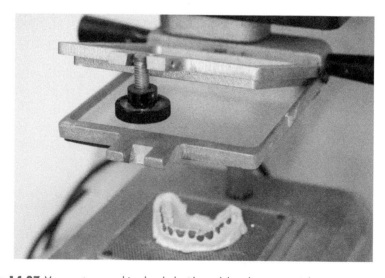

Figure 14.27 Vacuum tray machine loaded with model and tray material

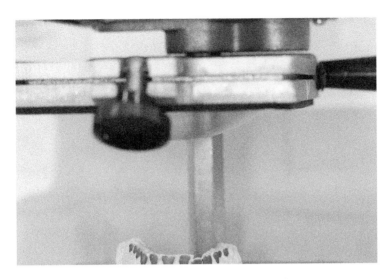

Figure 14.28 Warmed EVA sheet hanging below reservoir ready for use

INTRA- AND EXTRA-ORAL PHOTOGRAPHY

Photographs are an important diagnostic and assessment tool for the clinician, as well as being a powerful method of convincing patients that a dental problem exists or of showing them the before and after appearance of suggested dental treatments. Digital images in particular are extremely useful when a second opinion is required about a case (especially potentially suspicious soft tissue lesions), as they can be securely emailed to a specialist. Away from the hospital environment, photographs are used a great deal to assist in orthodontic assessments and to provide before and after views once orthodontic treatment has been completed. A suitably trained dental nurse can be tasked to take both intra- and extra-oral photographs for these purposes.

Old-style clinical photography involved the use of 'instamatic' type cameras, which produced a hardcopy 'polaroid' image within a few minutes. Digital imagery produces instant images without the need for film, and these can be loaded directly onto a computer and also downloaded as a hard copy if required. Once on the computer screen, they can be 'zoomed in' so that the image (or a section of it) can be enlarged, although the clarity of the picture deteriorates after a certain point.

An example of a suitable camera and attachments for clinical photography is shown in Figure 14.29.

The particular features of the camera and its potential uses are as follows:

- The camera body has interchangeable lenses, the one required for intra-oral (close up) photography is a macro lens
- The ring flash shown provides sufficient diffuse light directly at the object, rather than a bright burst of intense light in the surroundings as produced by an ordinary flash – it is simply screwed onto the camera body top and to the lens with a ring adapter
- The mode dial on top of the camera body allows the camera to automatically set itself to take images in the selected mode – so on this camera, close-up shots are taken with

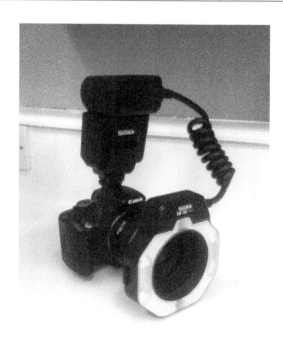

Figure 14.29 Digital camera with macro lens and ring flash

the dial set to the flower pictogram, while portrait images are taken with it set to the head pictogram (Figure 14.30)

- The lens focus mode switch on the side of the lens is used to change between automatic focus (AF) and manual focus (MF) – usually AF is used, but when intra-oral images are taken looking into the mouth, sometimes the camera automatically focuses onto the lip or an anterior tooth, when the image required is more posterior – in these cases, MF should be used and the lens focused manually by the operator onto the required focal point
- When taking intra-oral images, the soft tissues often need retracting either by hand, with a mouth mirror, or using specific lip retractors (Figure 14.31)
- Difficult-to-see areas such as the upper arch or lingual to the lower incisors can be viewed more easily with the use of oral mirrors (see Figure 4.9a) – these are best run under cold water before use to prevent them from misting while the patient breathes, or by asking the patient to hold their breath while the image is taken
- A typical portrait-style view shows the patient's head in a face-on position (see Figure 7.3a), while Figure 14.32 shows an intra-oral view of a prepared cavity in a tooth – the lens focus mode was set to MF to avoid the camera automatically focusing on the anterior teeth or surrounding structures
- Images can be viewed immediately on the camera viewer or loaded onto the computer for a larger and more detailed image
- The memory card from the camera is removed and inserted into the correct entry port of a card reader device – an adapter may be necessary for some card types (Figure 14.33)

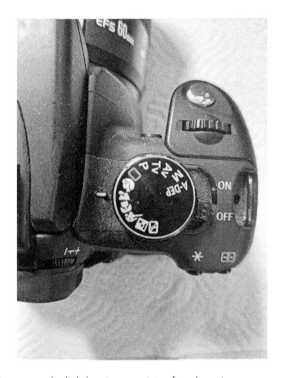

Figure 14.30 Camera mode dial showing a variety of mode options

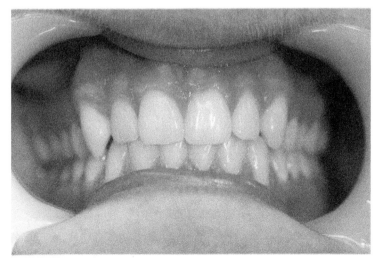

Figure 14.31 Use of lip retractors during intra-oral photography

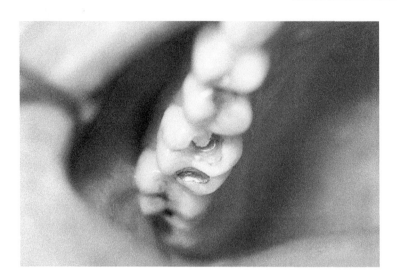

Figure 14.32 Use of manual focus to photograph a single tooth cavity

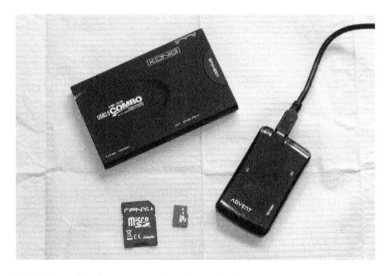

Figure 14.33 Examples of memory card readers and adaptors

- A USB cable connects the card reader to the computer and the images are present in the 'removable disk device' option – they can then be uploaded *en masse* as a file to the computer, or individually as a JPEG
- As the images are accessible immediately, any that require retakes can be carried out while the patient is still present

TAKING RADIOGRAPHS: PRESSING THE EXPOSURE BUTTON

While this task may seem a blatantly obvious skill to perform, the potential for harm to both the patient and the dental team from X-ray exposure if not carried out correctly has warranted its inclusion here.

During the taking of dental radiographs, whether intra- or extra-oral and digital or conventional, the moment at which the exposure button of the X-ray machine is pressed is the moment at which the X-ray beam is activated and fired at the patient and the X-ray film to produce an image. In the United Kingdom, the ability of the dental nurse to act as an operator during this procedure is entirely dependent on their being directly supervised by the 'set up' operator – the person who has positioned the patient and the film ready for the exposure. So, under no circumstances should any dental nurse without a post-registration qualification in dental radiography press the exposure button of any X-ray machine unless in the presence of another suitably qualified colleague. This also applies to the taking of test exposures for the purpose of quality assurance processes.

The exposure button itself is usually connected to the X-ray machine by an extendable electric cable so that the 'button pusher' can stand outside both the controlled area and the safety zone around the X-ray machine (Figure 14.34). The controlled area of a 1.5 metres radius from the machine head should only be occupied by the patient (and their carer or parent in certain circumstances), and the safety zone is deemed as another half metre outside this radius (so 2 metres in total), beyond which it is safe for the positioning of the dental team.

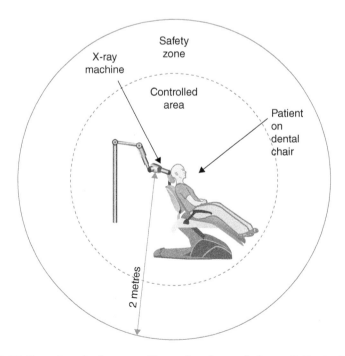

Figure 14.34 Illustration of safety zone (2 metres) and controlled area (1.5 metres) around the X-ray machine head

Beyond 2 metres, the potential amount of scattered radiation from the X-ray machine is considered negligible and the area is therefore safe. To ensure that this is the case, when significant dental exposures are undertaken in the workplace, the dental team wears personal dosimetry badges which are regularly analysed by specialists to ensure that no untoward X-ray exposures are occurring.

Procedure

Once a dental radiograph has been justified (it has been deemed necessary to be taken so that the clinician can make a diagnosis and/or provide dental treatment for a patient), the following actions will be carried out by the 'set up' operator:

- Film type and view chosen
- Patient and film positioned, using a film holder
- X-ray machine switched on and exposure time chosen (Figure 14.35)
- Check that everyone except the patient is outside the safety zone
- Verbal command given to the dental nurse operator to press the exposure button

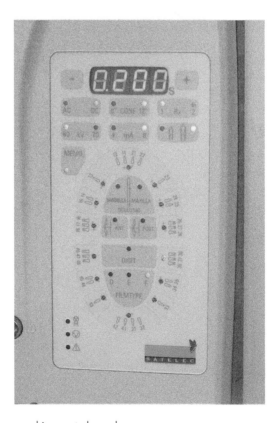

Figure 14.35 X-ray machine control panel

During the patient set-up and when instructed to do so by the 'set up' operator, the dental nurse operator will retrieve the exposure button device from the machine and move out to the safety zone (Figure 14.36). Modern dental X-ray machines will have audible buzzers that are activated during the exposure – some also have visible warnings of the exposure, such as illuminated signs or lights (Figure 14.37). When instructed to do so, and only then, the dental nurse operator will press and hold down the exposure button until the audible alarm stops. The button must not be pressed before requested as someone may still be within the controlled area or safety zone, while the button must not be released before the audible alarm stops as it is set as a timed exposure and an early

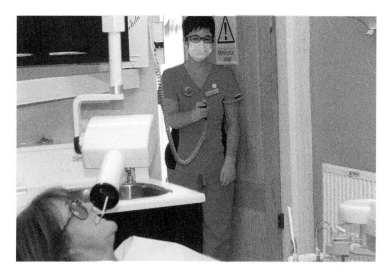

Figure 14.36 Dental nurse standing outside the safety zone with the exposure button

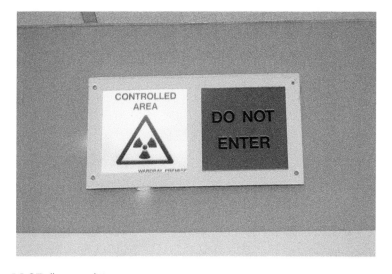

Figure 14.37 Illuminated X-ray warning sign

release will be too short to produce an image, the patient will have been exposed unnecessarily and the procedure will have to be repeated.

Very rarely a machine may malfunction – this is a potentially dangerous situation for the patient and the dental team, as X-ray over-exposure may occur. In this situation, the audible alarm may continue to buzz and the visible alarm may remain illuminated – it must be presumed under these circumstances that the machine is continuing to emit X-rays and must be shut down immediately. On instruction, the dental nurse operator must release the exposure button and remain outside the safety zone. The 'set up' operator has the responsibility of isolating the X-ray machine from the electrical supply or giving the command to do so, using the isolator switch located outside the safety zone – the presence of an isolator switch is a legal requirement under ionising radiation regulations. Once isolated, the machine must be marked as 'out of use', the patient must be informed of the situation, and the Radiation Protection Advisor and Medical Physics Expert must be notified of the error incident so that an investigation can be carried out. These actions are the responsibility of the 'set up' operator.

REMOVING SUTURES

Sutures are used to close a surgical site and hold the edges of a flap of soft tissue in position while the tissues heal, after surgery or trauma. Once the site has been checked by the dentist to ensure that full healing has occurred without any inflammation or infection present, the sutures can be carefully removed by a suitably trained dental nurse.

The procedure is often time consuming because care must be taken not to pull the healed surgical area as it will hurt the patient, and often there are several sutures to be removed.

The sterile instruments required for suture removal are a mouth mirror, a pair of college tweezers and either a pair of suture removal scissors or a disposable suture removal blade that can be loaded onto a standard scalpel handle (Figure 14.38). The scissors have

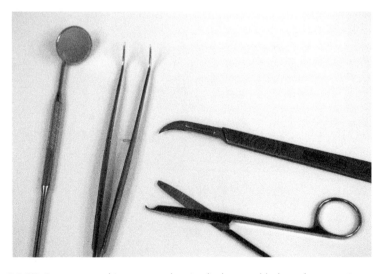

Figure 14.38 Suture removal instruments showing both suture blade and suture scissors

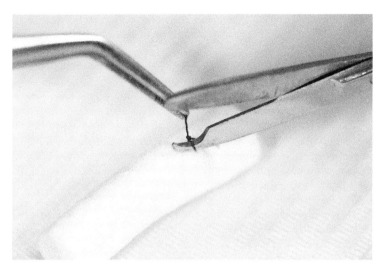

Figure 14.39 Holding suture end taut while cutting through the loop

a half-moon cut out of one blade so that the suture loop can be located here and held while being cut (Figure 14.39) – with an ordinary pair of scissors the loop would ride along the blade during cutting and pull uncomfortably on the wound. In Figure 14.39, the soft tissues are represented by a cotton wool roll so that the position of the suture loop in the scissor blade is more easily visible.

The technique of suture removal is as follows:

- The dental nurse and the patient wear appropriate personal protective equipment
- Angle the dental chair and light to provide easy access to the sutures
- Use the mouth mirror to retract soft tissues if necessary – sometimes a second dental nurse may be required to carry this out when the sutures lie posteriorly
- Remove any food debris from the sutures with a small-bore aspirator if necessary
- Count the number of sutures present and check with the procedure notes that they tally – if not, ask the patients if they were aware of losing any sutures (black braided silk is often used and may appear as a piece of black cotton to the patient) and refer back to the dentist for advice
- Gently find and hold one tied end of the suture with the tweezers, and then pull to hold it taut
- This should lift the top of the suture loop off the soft tissues, allowing the suture scissors to be placed beneath it with the cut out blade closest to the surgical tissues, or for the blade cutting edge to be placed in the same position when a suture removal blade is used rather than scissors
- The suture loop needs to be located in the half-moon cut out of the scissors blade so that the suture thread remains in place during cutting
- When correctly positioned, make the cut while holding the suture end with the tweezers
- Once cut through completely, the suture is removed from the mouth and placed on a tissue
- Repeat the process for all the sutures

- Count the number removed again, and then check that each one has been fully removed – they should each appear as a cut loop of thread with a knot and two tied ends present
- If any problems occur, seek the advice of the dentist – do not undertake any further tasks than the training allows

Post-operative advice

The patient should be advised to continue hot saltwater mouthwashes for the next few days to assist the area to heal completely now that the sutures have been removed. They can carry out their routine oral hygiene techniques in this area without fear of catching the sutures, and they can eat and drink as normal. They should not touch the area with their fingers, as they may introduce infection.

Overall, there are many opportunities for registered dental nurses to expand their skills in extended duties without having to undertake formal training to do so, and the acquisition of any of these skills will be of great value to any dental workplace. Relevant use of their Personal Development Plan in line with the GDC's enhanced CPD requirements will ensure that these extended duties remain current during the dental nurse's career, ensuring their respected position as a valued, worthwhile, and professional member of a modern dental team.

EXTENDED DUTIES OF THE DENTAL NURSE

Assessment sheets

Example of an oral hygiene instruction assessment sheet

PATIENT IDENTIFIER	2328
DATE	11th July 2023
REASON FOR OHI SESSION	Currently, no ID cleaning being carried out so several areas of tartar accumulation found at exam appointment
OHI AIDS USED	Tooth model, range of ID icon brushes, dental tape, wall mirror
COMMUNICATION SKILLS	Good, non-judgemental, helpful, keen to encourage patient to have a go with various aids used and congratulatory when successful
SPECIFIC ADVICE GIVEN	Sized patient for icon brushes – pink anteriorly and blue posteriorly, apply smear of toothpaste to brush before each insertion, wash brush after use, discard when looking worn
ABLE TO ANSWER PATIENT QUESTIONS	Yes – patient asked if she could just use pink brushes throughout, explained that they would be too small to clean wider contact areas for back teeth and therefore tartar likely to return here
ASSESSED BY	CH
SATISFACTORY OR NOT YET SATISFACTORY	Satisfactory
NOTES	Well prepared for session Good and confident use of aids Good communication skills with pleasant demeanour Knowledgeable of OHI topic

Basic Guide to Dental Procedures, Third Edition. Carole Hollins.
© 2024 John Wiley & Sons Ltd. Published 2024 by John Wiley & Sons Ltd.

Example of an impression-taking assessment sheet

PATIENT IDENTIFIER	1963
DATE	10th February 2022
REASON FOR IMPRESSION(S)	Upper tooth whitening tray
MATERIALS USED	Alginate and water
TRAY(S) USED	Upper boxed single-use tray – perforated
EQUIPMENT AND OTHER MATERIALS USED	Mixing bowl, spatula, water measure and scoop tray handle, disinfection and packaging items
MIX DETAILS AND TRAY LOADING	Smooth mix with no residual powder tray fully loaded from posterior edge forward, with full coverage and no excess material
ANY COMPLICATIONS	Pt wary of gagging, therefore nervous but compliant
QUALITY OF IMPRESSION	Correctly set throughout on removal, no air blows or defects Full arch recorded
ASSESSED BY	CH
POST-OPERATIVE CARE GIVEN	Pt congratulated Assisted with providing mouth rinse and carried out removal of material from around pt lips
DISINFECTION AND PACKAGING DETAILS	Rinsed in dirty sink Immersed in impression disinfectant solution for 10 minutes Rinsed and wrapped in damp gauze Sealed in air-tight bag with completed laboratory docket, marked as 'disinfected'
SATISFACTORY OR NOT YET SATISFACTORY	Satisfactory
NOTES	Fully prepared for procedure Good communication with pt throughout Good mixing and loading technique Correctly determined when impression had set Removed without tearing impression Good pt care afterwards Correct disinfection and packaging carried out

Example of a suture removal assessment sheet

PATIENT IDENTIFIER	1745
DATE	3rd January 2023
PREVIOUS SURGICAL PROCEDURE	Surgical extraction of grossly carious UR6 (16) Flap raised
SITE CHECKED BY	CH
INSTRUMENTS SET OUT	College tweezers, mouth mirror suture scissors
NUMBER AND TYPE OF SUTURES	3 black braided silk
PRESENTATION AT ROS APPOINTMENT	Site healed, no inflammation present Some food debris on suture ends
NOTES OF ROS PROCEDURE	Sutures aspirated with narrow bore to remove food debris and make ends clear End of each suture was found and gently held taut while sutures were cut and removed Assisted by the second nurse to retract right cheek
ANY COMPLICATIONS	None once retraction assistance provided
POSTOPERATIVE INSTRUCTIONS GIVEN	Pt told to carry out HSWMW again today to prevent soreness Pt told to carry out routine OHI in the area from now, and return if any problems before the pre-set review appointment next month
ASSESSED BY	CH
SATISFACTORY OR NOT YET SATISFACTORY	Satisfactory
NOTES	No problems with set-up Accurate observation of surgical area re-healing Handled instruments competently and realised assistance with retraction was required Did not proceed with ROS until happy with retraction and visibility

Glossary of terms

Abrasion cavity a self-inflicted worn area produced at the neck of a tooth by overvigorous toothbrushing

Abscess an accumulation of pus surrounded by inflamed tissue, usually occurring at the root end or in a periodontal pocket and classed as either acute or chronic

Acid etch an acidic material used in dentistry on the enamel of a tooth to chemically roughen it, allowing greater adhesion of some fillings and cements

Acute infection an infection of sudden onset, and therefore associated with pain and swelling

Aesthetics relating to a pleasing appearance, as in the aesthetics of a veneer for instance

Air abrasion a technique of stain removal from the tooth surface using a jet of abrasive particles fired under pressure from a specialised dental handpiece

Alginate a commonly used dental impression material derived from seaweed

Aligners a set of preformed, gum shield-like orthodontic devices which are worn sequentially to gradually allow tooth movement to occur, resulting in well-aligned dental arches

Amalgam a malleable filling material used to fill cavities in posterior teeth, and composed of various metal powders mixed with liquid mercury

Apex locator an electronic device used during root treatment to determine the full length of a root canal, by giving off a signal when the apex has been located

Apicectomy the surgical removal of a root apex and any associated pathology, and involving access to the root via the jaw bone

Articulating paper thin carbon paper used to detect high spots on new restorations, by being placed between the teeth and leaving coloured marks when the patient occludes

Articulator a three-dimensional jig device that mimics occlusion and jaw movements when a set of study casts are accurately placed within

Attrition a type of tooth wear (surface loss) that occurs when the teeth of both jaws are repeatedly rubbed together, as occurs when the patient clenches or grinds their teeth

Bitewing radiograph a posterior intra-oral radiographic view, taken to show interdental caries or restoration overhangs

Bonding the technique of 'glueing' the brackets and tubes of a fixed orthodontic appliance to the patient's teeth using special adhesive dental materials

Bone resorption the natural process that occurs to the jaw bones after tooth extraction, so that a smooth ridge contour is produced

Bracket a metal or ceramic component of a dental orthodontic fixed brace that is bonded to the tooth surface so that alignment forces can be applied to the tooth during treatment

Bridge a dental device used to replace a missing tooth (or teeth) by the construction and insertion of a device made up of several crowns (units) joined together in a single span

Basic Guide to Dental Procedures, Third Edition. Carole Hollins.
© 2024 John Wiley & Sons Ltd. Published 2024 by John Wiley & Sons Ltd.

Bruxism the habitual clenching and grinding of the teeth, often causing excessive tooth wear (attrition) or tooth fracture

Buccal surface the surface of the posterior (back) teeth closest to the cheeks

Calcium silicates a new range of materials used in deep cavities to protect the pulp and allow the tooth to heal in the hope of avoiding tooth death and root canal treatment

Calculus mineralised deposits of plaque that form at the gingival margins causing inflammation, it is also referred to as tartar

Canines the sharp 'fang' teeth of the dental arches, two in each arch

Caries a bacterial infection of the hard tissues of the teeth causing cavities, also referred to as tooth decay in lay terms

Cephalograph a specialist radiographic view used mainly in orthodontics to determine the severity of a patient's jaw discrepancies

Chronic infection an infection of very slow but persistent onset, and therefore usually painless

Composite a malleable filling material used to fill cavities in anterior and posterior teeth, and which gives a tooth-like appearance to the completed filling

Cone beam computerised tomography (CBCT) a 3-dimensional radiographic view of the jaws that is particularly used for implant treatment

Conscious sedation an anxiety control technique using the administration of drugs to relax the patient sufficiently for treatment to proceed, while they remain conscious (awake) throughout the procedure

Contact point the point at which two adjacent teeth are in contact with each other, where food debris often becomes lodged after a meal

Cotton wool roll/pledget roll or small ball of absorbent material used for moisture control during dental treatment

Crown a dental device used to cover the whole of a tooth with a pre-constructed 'cap' made of precious metals, porcelain or other ceramics to strengthen the remaining tooth structure or to improve the aesthetics

Demineralisation the action of acids on the tooth enamel to produce weakened areas that are more prone to carious attack

Dental care professional (DCP) the term used in the United Kingdom to describe all members of the dental team other than the dentist

Dental impression a device used to record the patient's tooth positions in the dental arch using an impression material in a tray, so that the set material remains accurate while a cast (study model) is made

Dental pantomograph (DPT) a radiographic view taken to show all of the teeth and their surrounding bony structures in one image, and used in orthodontics and complicated case diagnoses

Dentine the inner living tissue forming the bulk of the tooth structure, it contains nerve endings and therefore allows sensation in the tooth

Denture a removable oral device constructed from acrylic or chrome cobalt that is provided to replace one or more missing teeth in the dental arch

Disclosing tablet a coloured tablet of vegetable dye which stains plaque when chewed in the mouth; it is used during oral hygiene instruction to show patients where their plaque has accumulated and to assist them in its full removal

Distal surface the surface of any tooth which lies furthest away from the midline of the dental arch (the 'back' of the tooth)

Edentulous the condition of having no natural teeth present

Elevator a single-bladed surgical hand instrument used in dentistry to assist in tooth extraction

Enamel the outer surface of the erupted crown of a tooth, it is a mineralised, non-living tissue

Endodontics the branch of dentistry concerned with treatment involving the pulp tissue of the tooth

Erosion a type of tooth wear (surface loss) caused either by the excessive intake of dietary acids or by repeated exposure to acidic stomach contents, as occurs with gastric reflux or vomiting conditions such as bulimia

EVA tray material a sheet of a rubbery material used to create whitening trays and gum shields

Extended duties in the United Kingdom, those additional duties that may be performed by a dental nurse following appropriate and recorded training, over and above those skills acquired at basic certification

Extirpation the correct term for the removal of the pulp tissue from the tooth during endodontic treatment

Extraction of a tooth, the procedure of permanently removing a tooth from its socket

Fissure a natural anatomical cleft in the occlusal surface of a tooth, between the cusps

Fissure sealant a resin-like material used to seal over the tooth fissures and prevent food debris from lodging there and causing cavities

Floss or tape, a length of often waxed cotton-like material used to dislodge pieces of food debris from between the teeth

Fluoride a compound of the chemical fluorine which is added to oral health products (toothpaste, mouthwash and so on) to help prevent dental cavities from forming in the teeth

Forceps surgical instruments used to extract a tooth from its socket

Free sugars those sugars other than lactose which have been added to foods and drinks or are released during food processing, and that are responsible for causing tooth decay (previously referred to as non-milk extrinsic sugars)

Functional appliance a type of orthodontic appliance which corrects the position of the lower jaw using the muscular forces involved during the natural growth of the jaw

Gingival crevice a 2 mm deep crevice around the necks of all healthy teeth, where plaque accumulates when oral hygiene standards are poor

Gingival margin the edge of a restoration (such as a crown) that lies at the gingival crevice

Gingivitis inflammation of the gingivae, or gums

Glass ionomer a malleable dental material which can be used to fill cavities or cement items such as crowns, veneers and orthodontic brackets onto the teeth

Gutta percha point a natural rubber material used to root fill a tooth and provided in various length and diameter points

Haemostasis the arrest of blood flow in an area, especially after tooth extraction

Hidden sugars those sugars artificially placed into food products during manufacture that the consumer would not expect to be present in a particular item, especially those placed in savoury products

Immediate replacement denture a denture which is inserted at the time of tooth extraction, to replace missing teeth immediately

Impaction the prevention of a tooth from growing into its normal position in the dental arch due to crowding, or obstruction by either another tooth or the jaw bone

Implant a threaded titanium cylinder which is surgically screwed into the jaw bone to support an artificial tooth, teeth, or a denture; it is a method of tooth replacement

Incisor the four chisel-shaped biting teeth located at the front of each jaw

Inlay a solid dental device used to close a cavity in a tooth, using a material such as gold or porcelain and made out of the mouth by a technician

Intensifying screen a device used within extra-oral radiographic cassettes to reduce X-ray exposure to the patient

Interdental area the natural space that should be present between two adjacent teeth between their contact point and the gum margin

Intra-oral radiograph one that is exposed to X-rays while within the patient's mouth

Labial surface the outer surface of an anterior (front) tooth that lies against the lips

Lens focus mode switch a control button on a camera which allows the operator to choose between automatic focus (controlled by the camera) and manual focus (controlled by the operator) when taking intra- and extra-oral dental images

Lingual surface the inner surface of any lower tooth that lies against the tongue

Lining a material used in the base of a cavity before filling, to protect the underlying pulp tissue

Local anaesthetic a pharmaceutical that is injected in the mouth to anaesthetise (numb) a tooth or several teeth and their surrounding soft tissues, so that dental treatment can be carried out painlessly

Luting cement a cement mixed to a creamy consistency and used as an adhesive in crown and bridge cases

Malalignment the uneven, out-of-line positions of teeth in a dental arch, often caused by crowding

Mandible the anatomical term for the lower jaw

Mastication the correct term for the act of chewing of food

Matrix band a thin strip of metal or acetate used in a holder to separate adjacent teeth during filling

Maxilla the anatomical term for the upper jaw

Mesial surface the surface of any tooth which lies closest to the midline of the dental arch (the 'front' of the tooth)

Minor oral surgery a variety of surgical procedures carried out in the mouth which do not necessitate hospital admission, and which are usually carried out under local anaesthesia

Mode dial a control dial on a camera which can be altered by the operator for different types of photographic view (portrait, landscape, close-up, action and so on), which allows the camera to automatically set itself to take the ideal image for that particular setting

Moisture control the act of removing fluid contamination from the oral cavity during dental procedures, often involving the use of suction equipment and absorbent materials

Molar the largest of the teeth (up to six in each arch) which is located at the back of the mouth and is used for chewing and grinding food

Nitrous oxide or 'laughing gas', the anaesthetic gas used during inhalation sedation to reduce the anxiety level of the patient

Non-vital tooth one that has died

Obturation the correct term for the 3-dimensional sealing of a root canal during endodontic treatment, to prevent the future ingress of bacteria

Occlusal surface the biting surface of a posterior tooth

Occlusion the tooth positions achieved when the jaws are closed together and the upper and lower teeth are contacting

Oral health promotion the personalised information given to a patient to help them improve their own level of oral health

Oral hygiene instruction the practical methods and techniques demonstrated to a patient to help them improve their level of plaque removal from the teeth, so that their overall oral hygiene is improved

Orthodontics the branch of dentistry concerned with the correction of malocclusions and malalignment of teeth

Overdenture a denture constructed to attach to and fit over the top of implant abutments

Palatal surface that of all upper teeth that is closest to the roof of the mouth, rather than the lips or cheeks

Periapical radiograph an anterior or posterior radiographic view, taken to show a full tooth including its root and the bone immediately surrounding it

Periodontal disease (periodontitis) an infection of the supporting structures of a tooth in its socket, by one of several bacterial microorganisms, often referred to as 'gum disease' in lay terms

Periodontal ligament the tough connective tissue that holds a tooth in its socket

Personal protective equipment (PPE) items worn by the dental team and/or provided to the patient during dental treatment, which reduce the risk of contamination between staff and patients during the procedure (such as gloves, bibs, face masks)

Plaque a sticky film of food debris and bacteria (biofilm) that forms on the teeth causing caries and gingivitis if not removed

Plaque index a numerical score given to the presence of plaque in the patient's mouth at the time of checking, which is used to help monitor their oral hygiene levels before, during and after treatment

Premolar one of four teeth in each jaw which is located between the canine and first molar and is used for biting and chewing food

Post-operative instructions those given to a patient verbally and/or in writing after a dental procedure, to ensure that they come to no harm or do not compromise the success of the dental treatment they have just received

Pre-operative instructions those given to a patient (usually in writing) before a dental procedure, to ensure that they do nothing to compromise themselves or the success of the dental treatment they are about to receive

Probe a hand instrument of varying design, used during examination and diagnosis to detect either dental cavities in teeth, or periodontal pockets around teeth

Pulp chamber the inner hollow chamber of a tooth, containing nerve tissue and blood vessels (pulp)

Pulpectomy the removal of the whole tooth pulp from the entire pulp chamber; it is also referred to as root canal treatment or root canal therapy

Pulp exposure the breaching of the pulp chamber and exposure of its contents to the oral cavity

Pulpitis inflammation of the pulp tissue within a tooth

Pulpotomy the removal of the pulp tissue from the top of the pulp chamber only (the tooth crown), leaving that in the root of the tooth intact

Pulse oximeter a machine used to help monitor a patient during conscious sedation therapy, which records their oxygen saturation and pulse, and sometimes their blood pressure

Refined sugar a sugar not naturally present in food but added during manufacture, and highly cariogenic

Restorative dentistry the branch of dentistry usually involved with the restoration (filling) of teeth so that they are restored to full function and aesthetics

Root apex the very tip of a tooth root, where nerves and blood vessels enter and leave the tooth

Rubber dam a sheet of rubbery material used to isolate a tooth during dental procedures to provide good moisture control

Saliva the watery fluid naturally produced by the salivary glands and emptied into the oral cavity to provide lubrication, amongst other functions

Scaler an instrument used to remove calculus from teeth and roots

Sensitivity the term used to describe uncomfortable/painful sensations in the teeth when exposed to temperature extremes, especially to cold

Sensor (or receptor) the device used in digital radiography to capture an image when exposed to X-rays, rather than the film used in conventional radiography

Shade guide a collection of artificial tooth moulds in a range of colours from bright white to dark yellow, used by the dentist and technician to determine the required colour when constructing dentures or crowns, bridges and veneers

Short-term orthodontics a type of orthodontic treatment carried out for cosmetic reasons and usually only involving the anterior teeth, which can be completed in a much shorter time frame than conventional orthodontics

Stagnation area any area in the oral cavity that allows the accumulation of plaque to occur, either occurring naturally such as the fissures of the teeth, or such as overhanging filling edges

Stock tray a plastic or metal standard-shaped tray used for taking initial impressions or study model casts

Stomatitis inflammation of the mouth/oral soft tissues

Supine lying horizontal, as in the usual working position of the dental chair during procedures such as restorations

Suture the correct medical term for a 'stitch' – a piece of tied material (such as silk) which is used to hold the cut ends of a wound together while tissue healing takes place

Tartar the lay term for dental calculus

Tooth whitening the procedure of applying various chemicals to the teeth to lighten their intrinsic colour, either at the dental practice or using take-home kits

Topical anaesthetic a gel applied to the oral soft tissues to numb them before injecting a local anaesthetic

Vasoconstrictor a chemical added to local anaesthetic solutions to prolong anaesthesia by constricting the surrounding blood vessels

Veneer a dental device used as a 'false front' to a tooth, usually to hide discolouration or to alter the shape of a tooth

Wax bite rims laboratory constructed blocks of wax used during denture construction, that allow the dentist to record the correct occlusion of the patient so that the technician can place the denture teeth accurately

Xerostomia the correct term for the condition of 'dry mouth'

X-ray cassette a specialised case containing intensifying screens, used for extra-oral radiography such as orthopantomographs

Index

Basic Guide to Dental Procedures, Third Edition. Carole Hollins.
© 2024 John Wiley & Sons Ltd. Published 2024 by John Wiley & Sons Ltd.